A COLOR ATLAS OF
HEART DISEASE

A COLOR ATLAS OF HEART DISEASE

PATHOLOGICAL, CLINICAL AND INVESTIGATORY ASPECTS

George C. Sutton
Hillingdon Hospital, Middlesex, UK

Kim M. Fox
National Heart Hospital, London, UK

Contributors

John Bayliss
St Albans City Hospital, Herts, UK

John Swales
University of Leicester School of Medicine,
Leicester, UK

Foreword by

Desmond Julian
Consultant Medical Director
British Heart Foundation

J.B. LIPPINCOTT COMPANY *Philadelphia*

Acknowledgements

The authors are grateful to John Swales, Professor of Medicine, University of Leicester, for the chapter on Hypertension, and to John Bayliss, National Heart Hospital, and John Davies, Royal Gwent Hospital, for their help on the sections dealing with Heart Failure and Restrictive Cardiomyopathy, respectively. Many of the illustrations used in Chapter 3 on Hypertension were generously made available by Dr EH Mackay of Leicester General Hospital.

The authors gratefully acknowledge the contributions of Michael Davies, Simon Rees, Robert Anderson, Stuart Hunter, Ian Kerr, Graham Leech, Fergus McCartney, Michael Rigby and the authors, editors and contributors to the following publications:

The Slide Atlas of Cardiology and Supplement (Sutton, Anderson and Fox. Medi-Cine Ltd, 1978 and 1986)

Physiological and Clinical Aspects of Cardiac Auscultation (Harris, Sutton, Towers. Medi-Cine Ltd, 1976)

An Introduction to Echocardiography (Leech, Kisslo. Medi-Cine Productions, 1981)

An Introduction to Nuclear Cardiology (Walton, Ell. Current Medical Literature, 1985)

An Introduction to Cardiovascular Digital Subtraction Angiography (Hunter, Walton, Hunter. Current Medical Literature, 1987)

An Introduction to Magnetic Resonance of the Cardiovascular System (Underwood, Firman. Current Medical Literature, 1987)

In the preparation of this second edition, the authors wish to thank Dr John Cleland, Hammersmith Hospital, Dr David Hackett, Royal Postgraduate Medical School and Dr Richard Underwood, National Heart Hospital, for their meticulous review and constructive suggestions. In addition, they also wish to thank Dr Cleland for supplying figure 17 in Chapter 1, and Dr Underwood for supplying the illustrations used in the sections on Nuclear Techniques in Chapters 1 and 2.

Distributed in the USA and Canada by
J.B. Lippincott Company, East Washington Square,
Philadelphia, PA 19105, USA
Printed and bound in GB

© 1988, 1990 (revised edition) Current Medical Literature Ltd,
40–42 Osnaburgh Street, London NW1 3ND, UK

ISBN   0-397-58318-4

Library of Congress Catalog
Card Number 90-60687

Contents

Foreword

Once upon a time, doctors could learn all they wanted to know about cardiology from 'hands-on' experience. It was possible to acquire all the techniques available such as auscultation and electrocardiography without too much difficulty, and they could also spend time in the post-mortem room seeing the whole spectrum of the specialty. These days have gone — few if any cardiologists have command of all the technologies available today, and the post-mortem room is now seldom visited. Furthermore, the once common rheumatic and congenital heart diseases are seldom seen by the physician looking after adult patients and much learning has to be second hand. This being so, a good alternative to personal experience is to study outstandingly good illustrations such as those provided by this volume. Kim Fox and George Sutton, together with their collaborators, have put together a text and pictures which will go a long way to providing a valuable resource on cardiology for both teachers and students.

Professor DG Julian
Consultant Medical Director
British Heart Foundation

Chapter 1.
Ischaemic Heart Disease

Abbreviations

AMVL	Anterior Mitral Valve Leaflet	IVS	Interventricular Septum	N	Negative Contrast Effect
Ao	Aorta	LA	Left Atrium	PVW	Posterior Ventricular Wall
AoV	Aortic Valve	LAO	Left Anterior Oblique	RA	Right Atrium
AP	Antero-posterior	LAT	Lateral	RV	Right Ventricle
Eff	Effusion	LV	Left Ventricle	TV	Tricuspid Valve
		MV	Mitral Valve	VSD	Ventricular Septal Defect
		MVL	Mitral Valve Leaflet		

Note

The small images which accompany the text at the beginning of each chapter appear later in the chapter in a larger format.

2

Pathology

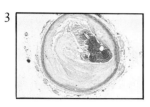

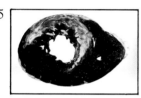

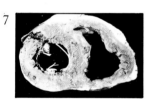

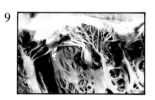

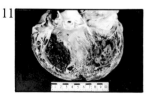

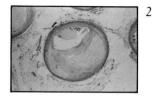

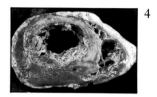

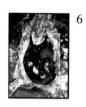

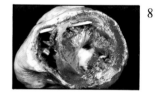

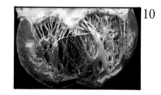

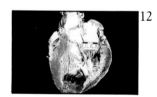

Patients with ischaemic heart disease almost always have atheroma of the coronary arteries [1] though episodes of myocardial ischaemia can occasionally result from spasm of normal coronary arteries. Rarer pathological lesions include coronary artery emboli or non-atheromatous disease of the coronary arteries or of the coronary ostia.

Although atheroma may occur to a variable extent in the coronary arterial tree, the histological pattern is consistent. Severe areas of stenosis show eccentric intimal thickening or plaques [2] containing large amounts of lipid. Lipid is often present as large pools of free cholesterol crystals separated from the lumen only by a thin layer of fibrous tissue. Thrombotic material is frequently present. Many areas of severe stenosis (>75%) have two or more lumina suggesting that they are recanalized total occlusions. Thrombotic total occlusions are due to a mass of fibrin and platelets plugging the lumen [3]. Calcification deep in the intima is common in atherosclerosis.

Although the initiating event causing myocardial infarction is unknown, plaque rupture leading to thrombosis of a coronary vessel may be important. This may lead to an area of muscle necrosis. The site of the infarct depends on the vessel involved. Thrombosis of the anterior descending coronary artery typically leads to an antero–septal infarct [4,5]. Disease in the right coronary artery results in a diaphragmatic infarct.

In transmural infarction, recent total occlusion due to thrombus in the supplying artery is invariably present [3]. Somewhat different pathological changes may be found when the infarct is non-transmural. These consist of sub-endocardial and focal areas of necrosis scattered throughout the ventricle. Occlusive thrombi are less consistently found.

Complications of acute myocardial infarction include rupture of the left ventricle into the pericardium [6,7], ruptured interventricular septum [8], ruptured papillary muscle [9], ischaemic papillary muscle resulting in severe mitral regurgitation [10], and formation of mural thrombus within the ventricles [11,12]. Later complications include the formation of a localized left ventricular aneurysm and dilatation of the left ventricle including areas of scarring [12].

Presentation

Symptoms

Patients with ischaemic heart disease may be asymptomatic in spite of widespread severe coronary atheroma. In contrast, other patients may die suddenly without extensive disease. The usual clinical presentation includes angina, acute myocardial infarction and heart failure. Some patients may present with arrhythmias (including sudden death) without any previous symptoms due to ischaemic heart disease.

Chest pain due to myocardial ischaemia typically occurs on physical exercise or during stress probably due to myocardial oxygen demand exceeding the coronary blood supply. Episodes of chest pain may also occur at rest. Such episodes may be due to a

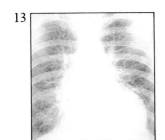

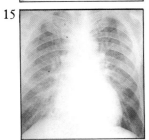

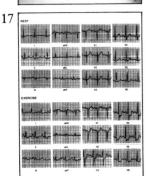

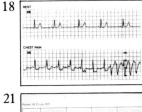

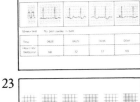

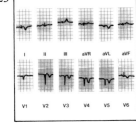

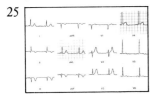

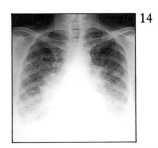

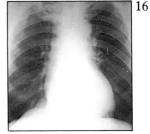

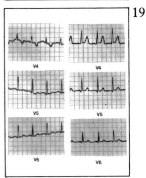

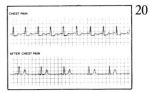

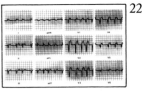

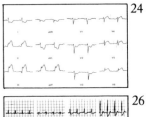

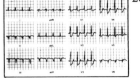

sudden reduction in oxygen delivery to the myocardium (eg. coronary artery spasm).

Patients whose symptoms appear to be stable may develop more readily provoked pain and episodes of pain that are entirely unprovoked. Occasionally such symptoms in some patients precede the development of acute myocardial infarction, while in others the unprovoked episodes fade and the patient often returns to, or establishes, a stable pattern of chest pain.

Many patients develop myocardial infarction without premonitory symptoms. Prolonged severe chest pain is a characteristic feature. The acute development of breathlessness following infarction may be due to extensive myocardial necrosis with resulting pulmonary oedema or rarely rupture of the ventricular septum or a papillary muscle. Arrhythmias are very common in acute infarction and may be asymptomatic or result in acute breathlessness or further chest pain or syncope.

Patients with chronic ischaemic heart disease may develop heart failure without recent myocardial infarction. Such patients may have either a localized left ventricular aneurysm or left ventricular dilatation with widespread areas of scarring resulting in severely compromised left ventricular function.

Signs

Many patients with chronic ischaemic heart disease do not have any abnormal physical signs. If there is left ventricular dysfunction, a double apical impulse will frequently be palpated and a fourth heart sound may be heard. In some patients with severe left ventricular disease, a loud pulmonary valve closure sound will be heard suggesting pulmonary hypertension. There may be a pansystolic murmur either due to chronic papillary muscle dysfunction with resultant mitral regurgitation or due to tricuspid regurgitation in patients with severe chronic heart failure with fluid retention. A third heart sound may be heard either in the patient with chronic severe ventricular dysfunction or in the acute phase of myocardial infarction with severe heart failure. The development of a pansystolic murmur shortly after acute myocardial infarction would suggest ischaemic damage to a papillary muscle, rupture of the ventricular septum or rupture of the papillary muscle. In patients with severe heart failure sinus tachycardia is common with summation of third and fourth heart sounds giving rise to the gallop rhythm. Reduced cardiac output, either as an acute or chronic complication, results in reduced perfusion of vital organs with consequent oliguria and renal failure, confusion due to poor cerebral perfusion and peripheral vasoconstriction.

Investigations

Radiology

Most patients presenting with angina in the absence of left ventricular dysfunction have a normal plain chest radiograph. With long standing generalized left ventricular dysfunction or a localised left ventricular aneurysm there may be cardiomegaly and features of pulmonary venous hypertension. In about 50% of

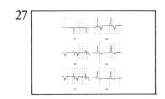

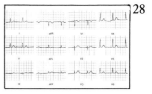

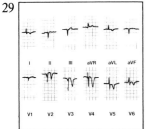

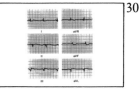

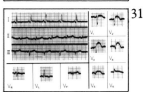

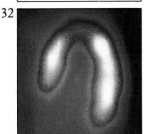

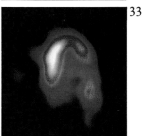

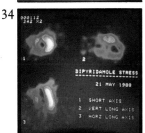

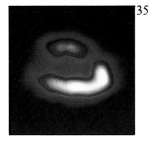

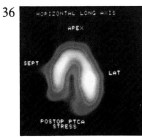

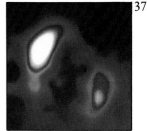

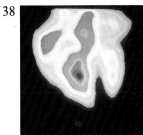

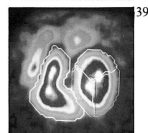

patients with a localized left ventricular aneurysm, the aneurysm may be visible on the radiograph as an abnormal bulge on the left heart border [13]. Pulmonary oedema may develop in the patient with chronic ischaemic heart disease or may follow acute myocardial infarction or one of its complications [14], such as ruptured interventricular septum or mitral regurgitation. In ruptured ventricular septum the pattern of pulmonary vessels sometimes suggests a left to right shunt [15,16].

Electrocardiography

The resting ECG may often be normal. However, it may show evidence of an old myocardial infarction, ST-T abnormalities, or left bundle branch block.

The electrocardiogram recorded during exercise is likely to show ST-segment abnormalities. The most specific change is down sloping ST-segment depression particularly in association with the development of chest pain [17]. Usually 1mm ST-segment depression is suggestive of myocardial ischaemia. The ST-segment may be upsloping, horizontal or down-sloping. Occasionally arrhythmias are recorded in association with ST-segment changes during exercise [18]. The presence of an abnormal resting ECG, particularly left bundle branch block, makes interpretation of ST-segment changes difficult.

During episodes of chest pain due to myocardial ischaemia, the 12 lead ECG is likely to show ST-T wave changes that resolve when the pain is relieved [19]. The rare patient with angina due to coronary artery spasm with or without coronary atheroma (Prinzmetal's angina) shows striking ST-segment elevation during an episode of chest pain [20].

Ambulatory monitoring of ST-segments in patients with ischaemic heart disease will often show ST-T wave changes during episodes of chest pain; frequently, however, such ECG changes may be recorded in the absence of chest pain [21] and are also likely to be due to myocardial ischaemia.

Patients who have acute myocardial infarction usually show pathological Q waves and ST-T abnormalities which evolve with time. The location of the infarct can be roughly determined from the electrocardiogram; thus an acute anterior infarct shows Q waves and ST-elevation in the anterior precordial leads (V1 to V4) with similar changes in leads 1, AVL and V5 to V6 [22]. As time passes the ST-T changes evolve into T wave inversion [23]. More localized ECG changes are seen in septal (V2-V4) or lateral (I, AVL, V5, V6) infarction. An inferior infarct shows similar changes in the inferior leads (2,3 and AVF) [24,25]. A true posterior infarction shows dominant R waves in V1 reflecting the absence of posterior forces [26].

When the infarct is non-transmural (subendocardial) Q waves are not seen but there are usually striking ST-T changes which may resolve with time [27,28].

Patients with rupture of the ventricular septum following myocardial infarction usually show electrocardiographic features of a septal infarct [29] whereas those with papillary muscle infarction or ischaemia resulting in mitral regurgitation often show evidence of infero-lateral infarction [30]. These electrocardiographic features may help in distinguishing these two complica-

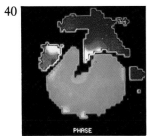

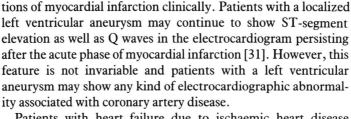

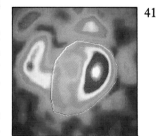

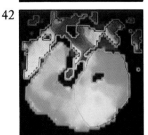

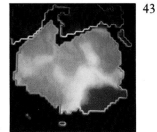

tions of myocardial infarction clinically. Patients with a localized left ventricular aneurysm may continue to show ST-segment elevation as well as Q waves in the electrocardiogram persisting after the acute phase of myocardial infarction [31]. However, this feature is not invariable and patients with a left ventricular aneurysm may show any kind of electrocardiographic abnormality associated with coronary artery disease.

Patients with heart failure due to ischaemic heart disease almost always have ECG evidence of previous myocardial infarction, ST-T wave abnormalities or left bundle branch block at rest.

Nuclear Techniques

Nuclear techniques show functional information which complements the anatomical information provided by, for instance, coronary arteriography. Thallium-201 is an isotope that is actively taken up by myocardial cells in proportion to myocardial perfusion. Subsequent imaging therefore provides a map of myocardial perfusion with defects representing areas either with impaired perfusion or with cellular ischaemia. The isotope is normally given at peak exercise with imaging immediately afterwards and again following a variable period of redistribution. Areas of infarction have reduced uptake in both images, but reversibly ischaemic myocardium has impaired uptake initially and improved uptake at rest. It is therefore possible to define normally perfused [32], reversibly ischaemic [33], and infarcted myocardium, and to assess the site and extent of abnormalities. The importance of such an assessment lies in the fact that the likelihood of future cardiac events is closely related to the extent of ischaemia. It is therefore possible to select patients at high risk, independently of coronary anatomy, and to concentrate revascularization procedures in this subgroup [34–36]. Planar images have traditionally been used, but a significant advance has been the use of rotating gamma cameras to acquire images from many angles from which to reconstruct emission tomograms. The three dimensional view of myocardial perfusion provided by tomographic imaging greatly increases the accuracy of assessment and hence the clinical value of the technique. A further development that has increased the scope of the technique is the use of intravenous dipyridamole, a coronary arterial dilator, to induce abnormalities of thallium uptake in patients with coronary artery disease without the need for dynamic exercise [37].

The second important nuclear cardiological procedure is radionuclide ventriculography using technetium-99m to label the intracardiac blood pools. Imaging is either performed during the first passage of the bolus through the central circulation or when it has reached equilibrium [38]. Left ventricular volumes, ejection fraction and parameters of diastolic function such as filling rates can be measured. Regional wall motion can also be assessed and helpful methods of displaying both the extent and the timing of contraction are the Fourier amplitude and phase images [39–42]. The phase image is particularly helpful in defining areas of dyskinesis suggesting left ventricular aneurysm [43]. Imaging during stress allows the response to exercise to be measured and a fall in LVEF and/or new regional wall motion abnormalities are suggestive of exercise induced ischaemia [44,45]. The LVEF during peak

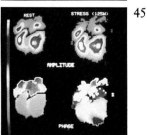

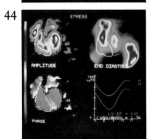

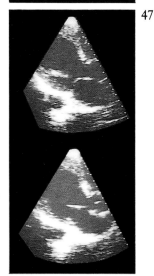

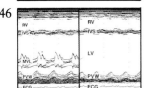

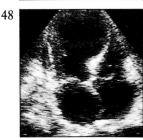

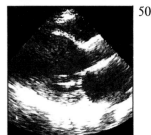

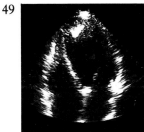

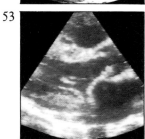

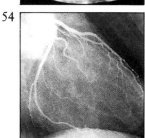

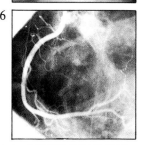

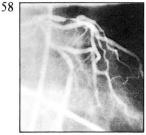

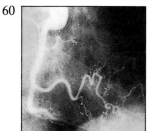

stress is, like the extent of ischaemia shown by thallium imaging, a powerful prognostic indicator.

Echocardiography

In patients with ischaemic heart disease and normal resting left ventricular function the echocardiogram is usually normal except in the rare circumstances where a recording is made during chest pain when regional wall motion abnormalities may be detected by 2-dimensional echocardiography. In those patients with chronic ischaemic heart disease who have abnormal left ventricular function, this may be detected by various techniques using echocardiography. M-mode echocardiography may show an increase in left ventricular dimension and reduction of wall motion when left ventricular disease is severe and generalized [46]. Sometimes, an M-mode echocardiogram showing lack of motion of either the septum or posterior wall will indicate permanent damage or scarring in those regions. 2-Dimensional echocardiography may visualize regional abnormalities within the overall function of the ventricle. Cases of extreme systolic wall thinning and/or dyskinesia are readily apparent from inspection of the systolic and diastolic images [47]. A localized left ventricular aneurysm may be detected by 2-dimensional echocardiography [48]. Thrombus within an abnormal ventricle may sometimes be seen [49].

In acute myocardial infarction, M-mode echocardiography may show outward movement of the endocardium during systole of either septum or posterior wall due in part to a reduction in wall thickness of either of these affected regions. 2-Dimensional echocardiography is usually superior in locating and determining the extent of infarcted myocardium [50].

Complications of acute myocardial infarction such as the development of a pericardial effusion [51], rupture of the ventricular septum resulting in a ventricular septal defect [52] and rupture of a papillary muscle causing flail-like motion of mitral valve leaflets may be identified using 2-dimensional echocardiography [53].

Cardiac Catheterization and Angiography

Although left ventricular pressures are often normal the most likely haemodynamic abnormality in patients with chronic ischaemic heart disease is an elevation of left ventricular end-diastolic pressure. This occurs most frequently if there is extensive chronic damage of the left ventricle or during an episode of myocardial ischaemia. In acute myocardial infarction, left ventricular end-diastolic and pulmonary capillary wedge pressure may be elevated and cardiac output reduced.

If the myocardial infarct is complicated by ventricular septal rupture, a left-to-right shunt at ventricular level will be demonstrated often with significant pulmonary hypertension. If the infarct is complicated by significant mitral regurgitation, the left atrial or pulmonary capillary wedge pressure will show a high 'V' or systolic wave. Cardiac output is likely to be reduced with either of these complications. In order to demonstrate the exact pattern of coronary artery narrowing coronary arteriography is required [54–60]. This technique may be required either in the patient

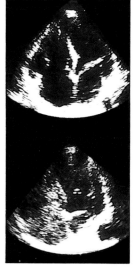

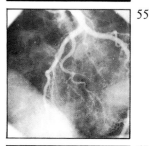

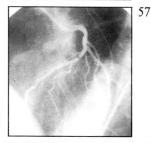

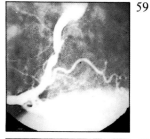

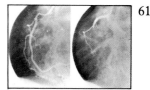

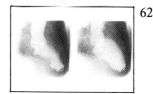

63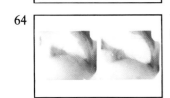

64

with chronic ischaemic heart disease or in the acute phase of myocardial infarction. The absence of angiographically demonstrable coronary artery narrowing does not exclude the possibility of the patient having transient myocardial ischaemia. Occasionally patients with normal or near normal coronary arteries may develop coronary spasm [61].

Left ventricular angiograms may demonstrate local [62] or generalized abnormalities of left ventricular contraction, localized left ventricular aneurysm [63], mitral regurgitation [64], and ruptured septum [65].

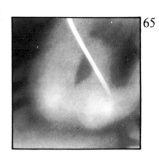 65

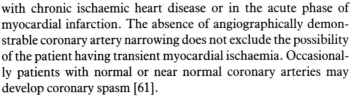

1   Longitudinal slice of coronary artery showing at least 80% narrowing of the lumen.

Anterior Descending Coronary Artery

Site of Narrowing

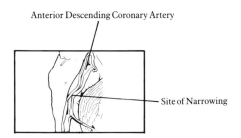

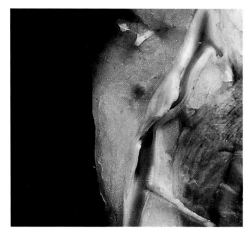

2   Narrowed coronary artery due to atherosclerosis - transverse section. The lumen is reduced to a small rather crescentic opening by a mass of intimal fibrous tissue containing lipid.

Lumen

Intimal Fibrous Plaque

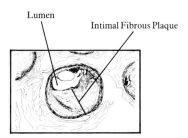

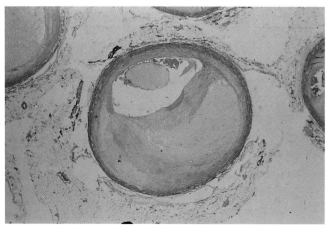

3   Thrombosed coronary artery in transverse section. The lumen is completely occluded by a mass of red thrombus. Above and to the left of the thrombus is a plaque of atheroma which contains lipid.

Lipid in Athermatous Plaque

Thrombus

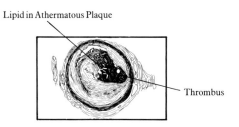

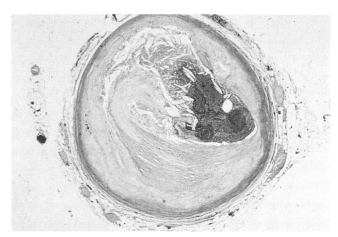

4   Transverse slice (fresh) of the ventricles. A recent (four day old) full-thickness myocardial infarction is present in the anterior wall of the left ventricle which extends into the interventricular septum.

Infarction

Interventricular Septum

Left Ventricle

Right Ventricle

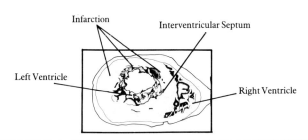

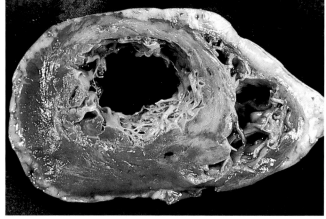

5 Slice of the ventricles stained to show succinic dehydrogenase enzyme activity (dark). An acute infarct is demonstrated as a white area due to the loss of enzyme activity.

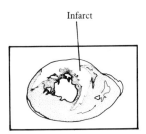

Infarct

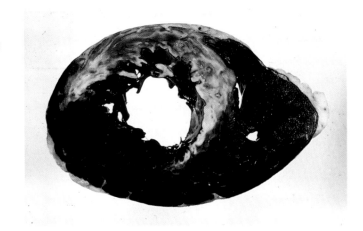

6 Pericardial sac filled with blood clot as a result of cardiac rupture due to myocardial infarction.

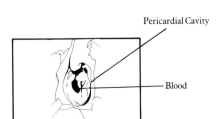

Pericardial Cavity

Blood

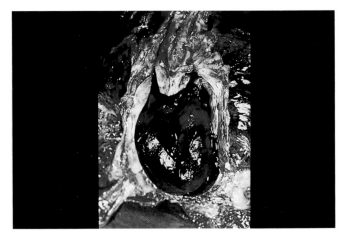

7 Rupture of the anterior wall of the left ventricle due to acute infarction.

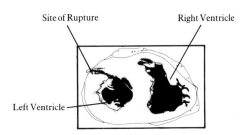

Site of Rupture   Right Ventricle

Left Ventricle

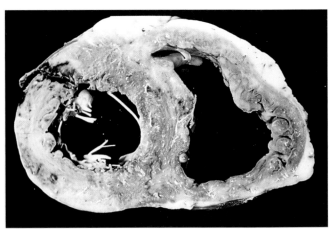

8 Acute myocardial infarction of the septum with rupture resulting in a ventricular septal defect (probe is shown passing through the defect).

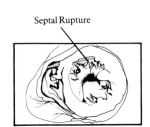

Septal Rupture

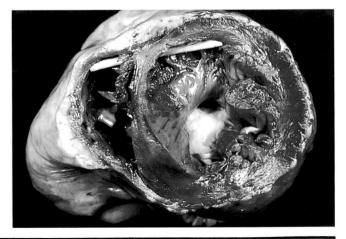

9 Acute myocardial infarction resulting in rupture of a papillary muscle.

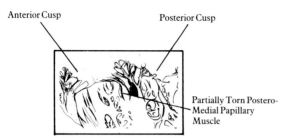

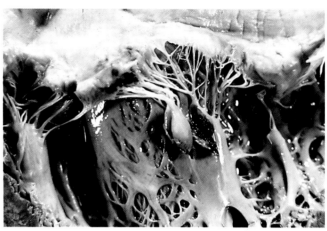

10 The left ventricle has been opened to show a papillary muscle infarct resulting in mitral regurgitation. The posterior papillary muscle is pale and shrunken due to infarction. The anterior papillary muscle (normal) is larger and darker. Subendocardial ischaemic scarring is present in the left ventricle.

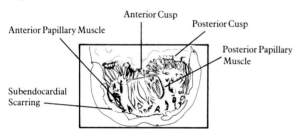

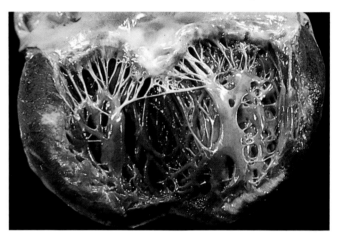

11 Widespread ischaemic scarring of the myocardium producing a dilated thin-walled ventricle. A thrombus has formed in one area in relation to the aneurysmal bulge of the ventricular wall.

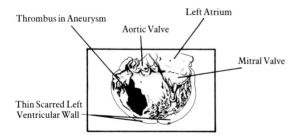

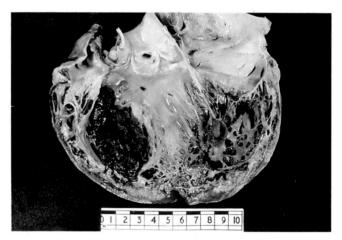

12 Localized left ventricular aneurysm due to ischaemic damage. The aneurysm does not contain more than a fine deposit of thrombus and has a larger central cavity opening into the ventricle.

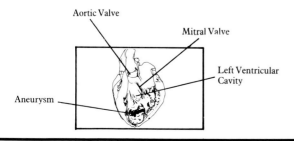

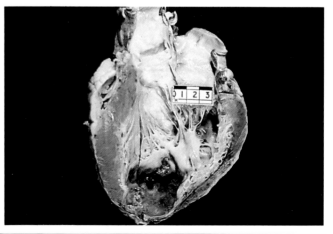

13 Chest radiograph showing an abnormal bulge on the left heart border due to a ventricular aneurysm. There is pulmonary oedema.

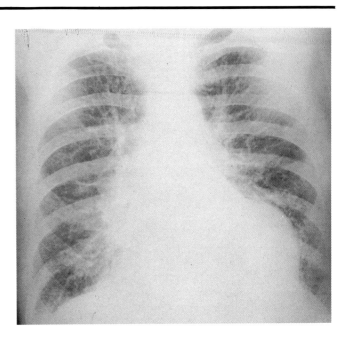

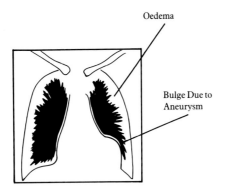

14 Chest radiograph showing pulmonary oedema and bilateral pleural effusions following acute myocardial infarction.

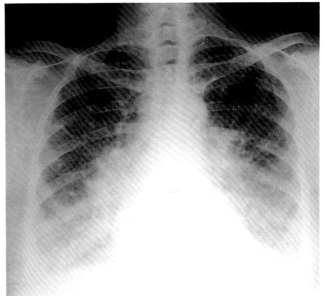

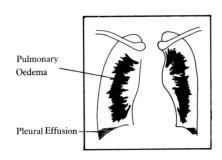

15 Chest radiograph showing cardiac enlargement with hilar oedema and generalized increase in pulmonary vessel size due to left-to-right shunt through a ventricular septal defect complicating myocardial infarction.

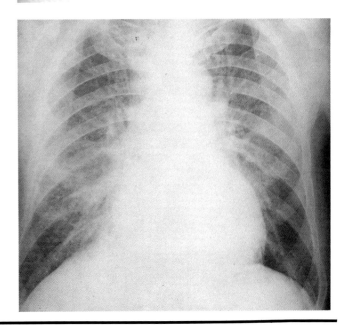

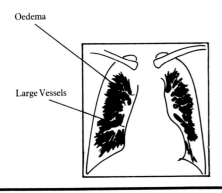

16 Chest radiograph of the same patient as [15] showing normal pulmonary vascularity following surgical closure of the defect.

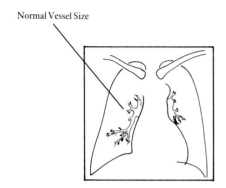

Normal Vessel Size

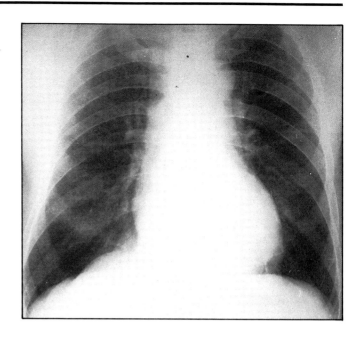

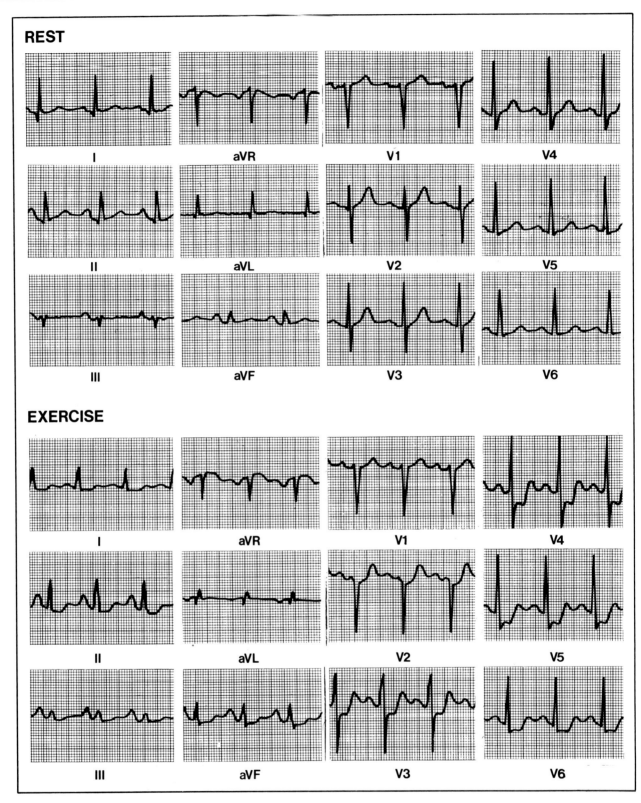

Resting and exercise electrocardiograms in a patient with angina. The resting electrocardiogram is normal. On exercise there is both horizontal and down sloping ST segment depression in the anterior chest leads associated with the development of chest pain.

18

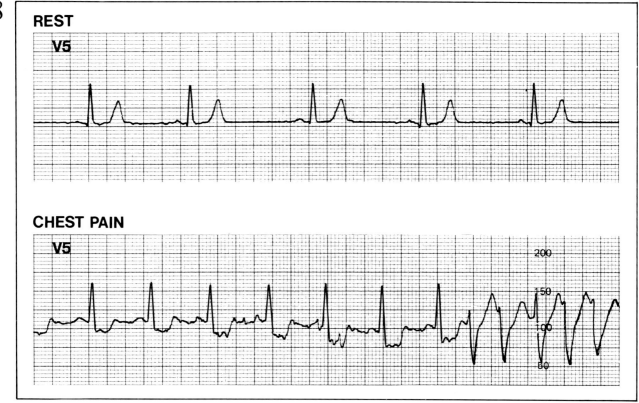

Electrocardiogram recorded during 24-hour ambulatory monitoring showing ST depression and the development of ventricular tachycardia during chest pain.

19

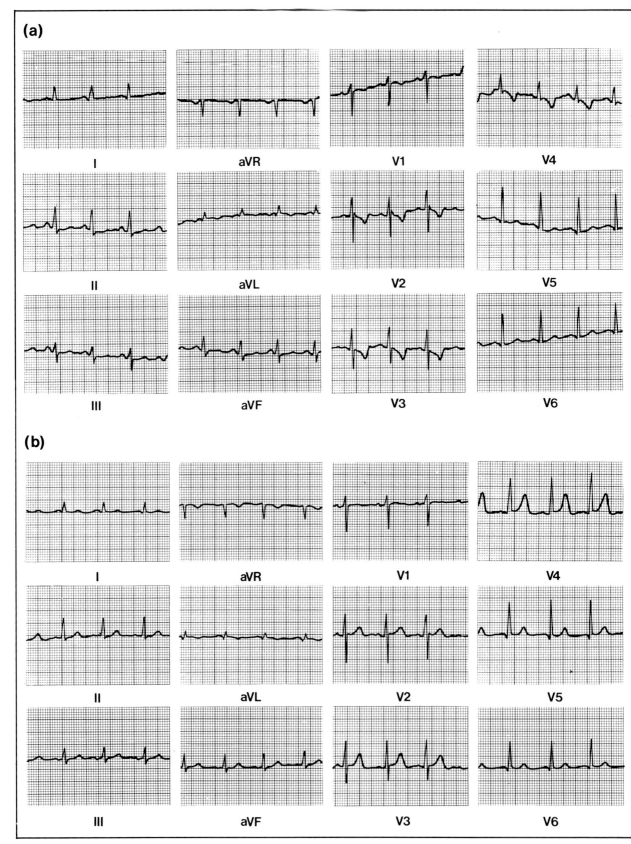

Resting electrocardiograms taken during chest pain in a patient with ischaemic heart disease showing ST-T wave abnormalities in the anterior chest leads (a). After the pain has subsided the ST-segment changes return to normal (b).

20

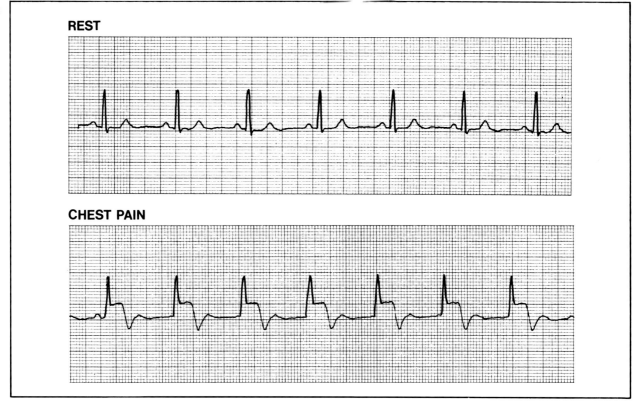

Electrocardiogram recorded during ambulatory monitoring showing ST-segment elevation during chest pain.

21

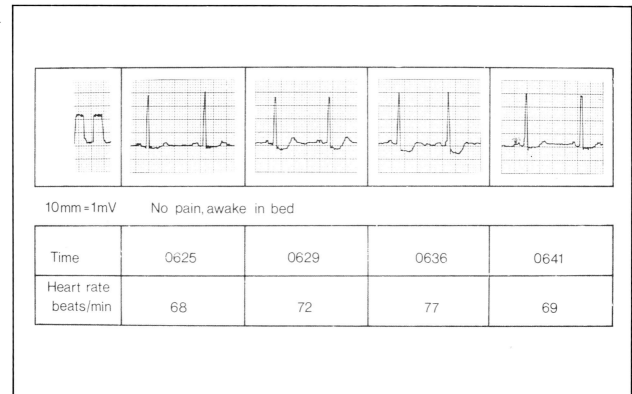

10mm = 1mV	No pain, awake in bed			

Time	0625	0629	0636	0641
Heart rate beats/min	68	72	77	69

Electrocardiogram recorded during 24-hour monitoring. There are transient ST-segment changes whilst the patient was lying awake in bed. He did not complain of chest pain.

22

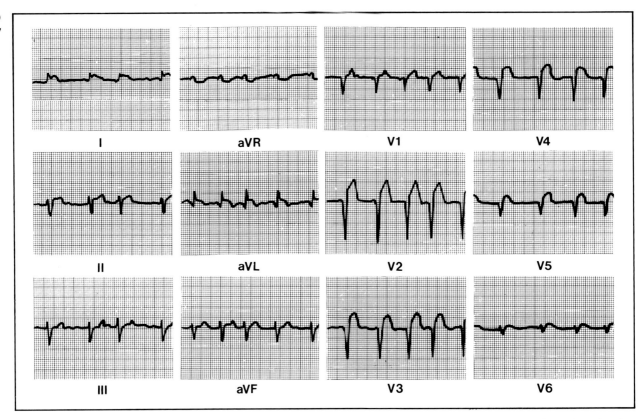

Electrocardiogram in a patient with acute antero-lateral myocardial infarction showing Q waves and ST elevation in V2-V5, I and aVL.

23

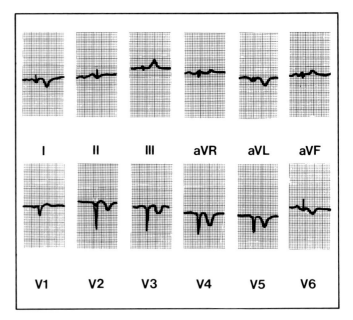

Electrocardiogram in the same patient as [22] taken several days later, showing T wave inversion in leads previously showing ST elevation with persisting Q waves.

24

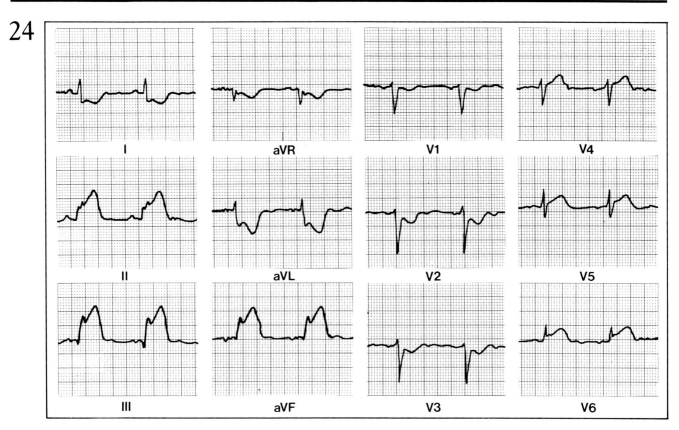

Electrocardiogram showing acute inferior myocardial infarction with ST elevation in II, III and aVF. There is also ST elevation in V5 and V6 and ST-segment depression in I, aVL, V2 and V3.

25

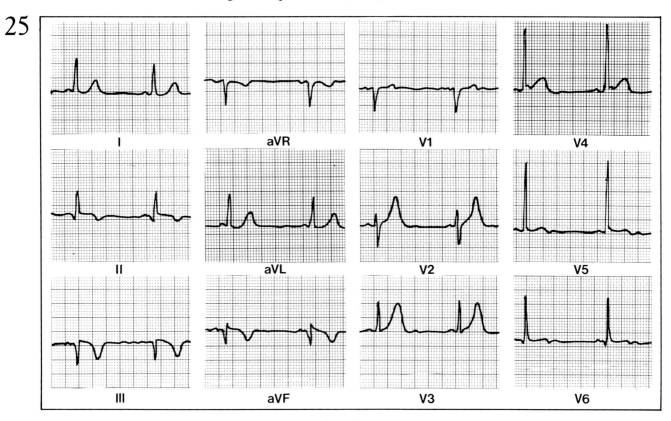

Electrocardiogram from the same patient as [24] showing Q waves and T wave inversion in leads II, III and aVF.

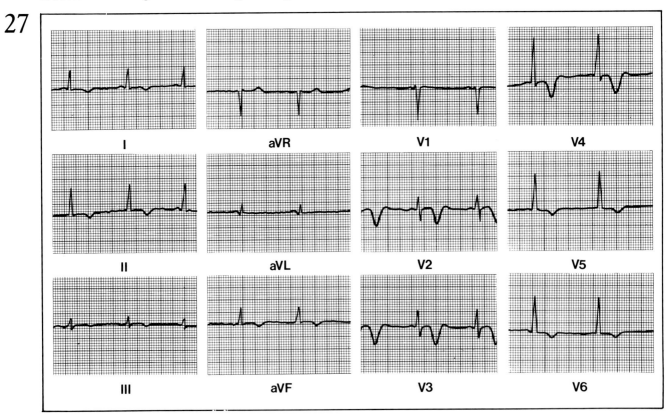

26

Electrocardiogram showing a true posterior myocardial infarction. There are Q waves in II, aVF and V6 with dominant R waves in V1-V4 together with ST-segment depression in the anterior chest leads.

27

Electrocardiogram from a patient with a subendocardial infarction showing widespread T wave inversion.

28

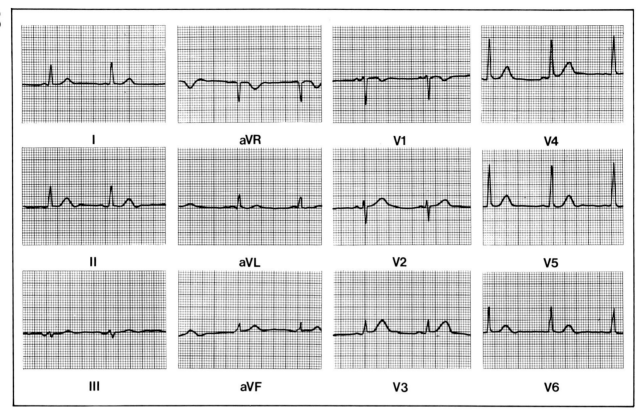

Electrocardiogram from the same patient as [27] several months later showing resolution of the T wave changes.

29

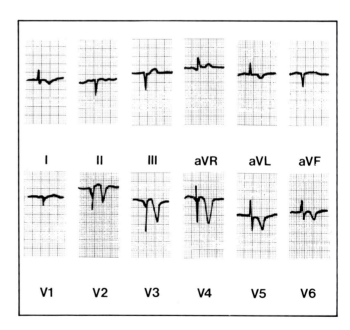

Electrocardiogram from a patient with a ruptured ventricular septum following myocardial infarction. There are Q waves in leads V1–V3 indicating septal infarction.

30

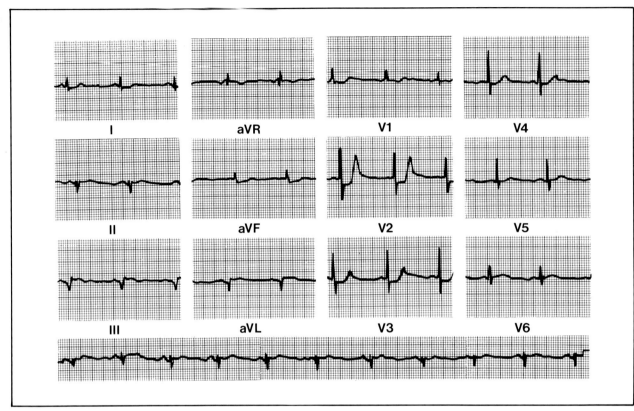

Electrocardiogram from a patient with mitral regurgitation secondary to inferior myocardial infarction. There are Q waves in the inferior leads, and incomplete right bundle branch block. The changes of true posterior infarction are also present.

31

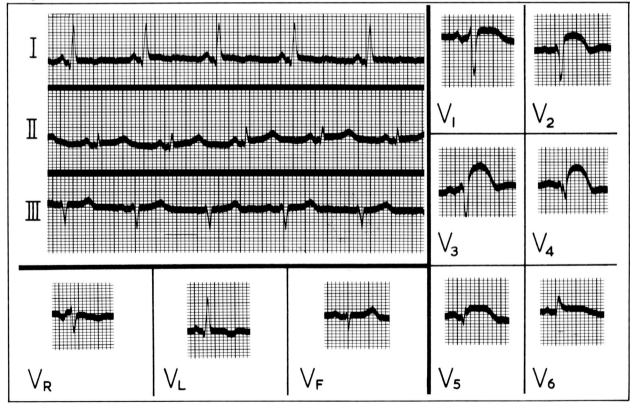

Electrocardiogram from a patient with a left ventricular aneurysm. There are Q waves and ST-segment elevation in the anterior leads some months following acute infarction.

32 Normal emission tomograms in vertical (top) and horizontal long axis (middle) and short axis planes (bottom). There is uniform uptake of thallium-201 throughout the myocardium.

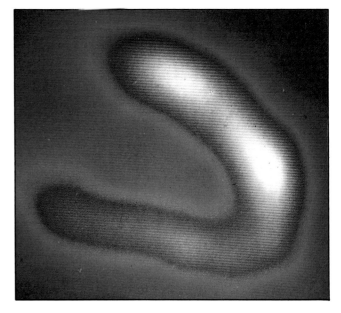

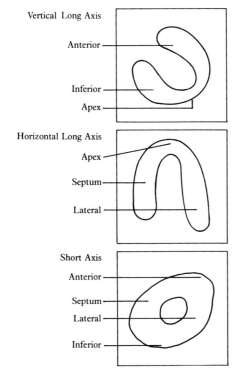

Vertical Long Axis

Anterior

Inferior

Apex

Horizontal Long Axis

Apex

Septum

Lateral

Short Axis

Anterior

Septum

Lateral

Inferior

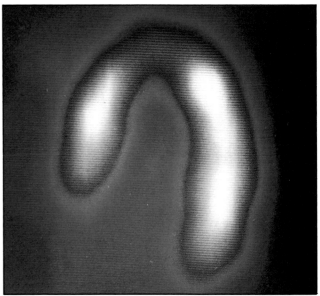

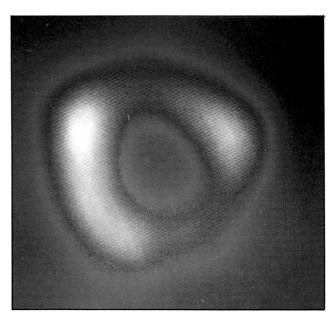

33

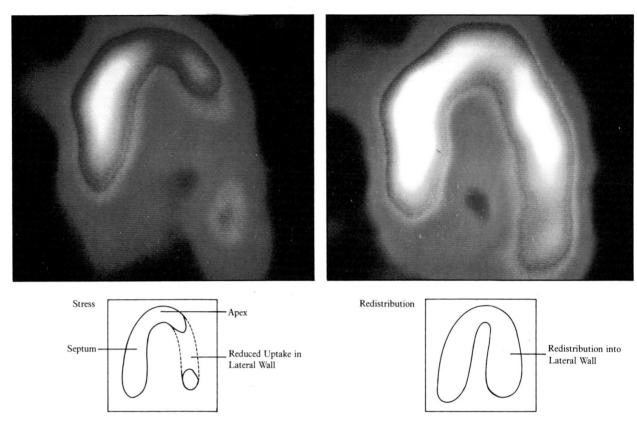

Stress (left) and redistribution (right) horizontal long axis tomograms showing reversible lateral wall ischaemia in a patient with left circumflex coronary artery disease.

34

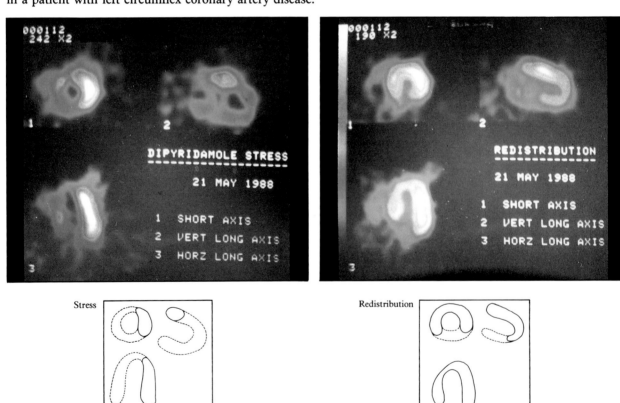

Stress (left) and redistribution (right) tomograms showing inferior infarction and reversible anteroseptal and apical ischaemia. This is a high risk scan because of the extent of ischaemia.

35

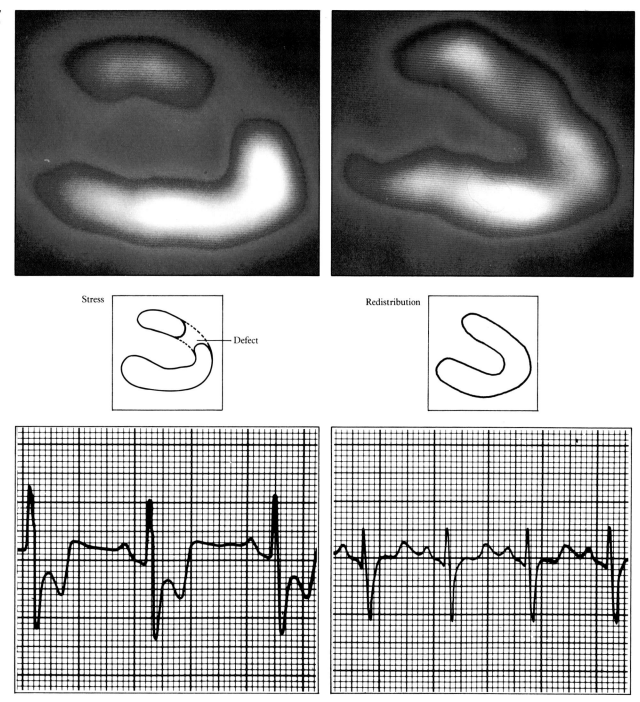

Stress (left) and rest (right) vertical long axis tomograms (top) and ECG (bottom) showing reversible anterior ischaemia. Because of the limited area of ischaemia, this is a low risk scan.

36

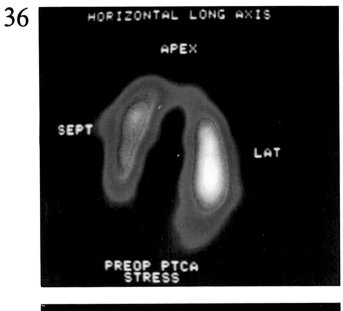
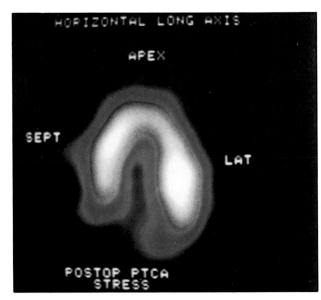
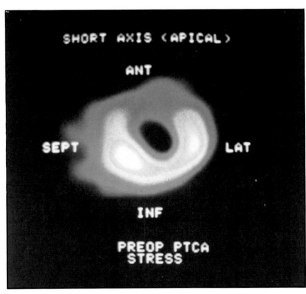
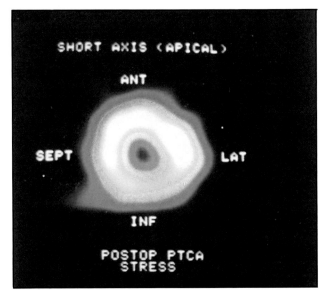
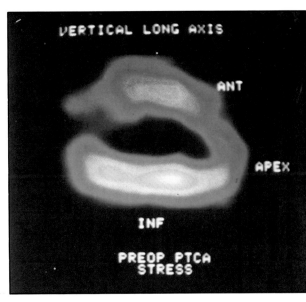
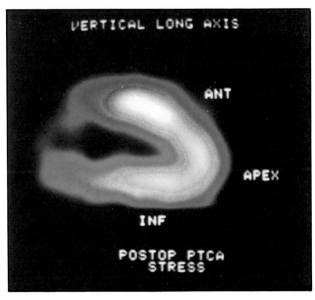

Stress tomograms before (left) and after (right) angioplasty to a left anterior descending lesion after the first septal branches. The small distal anterior area of ischaemia is abolished.

37

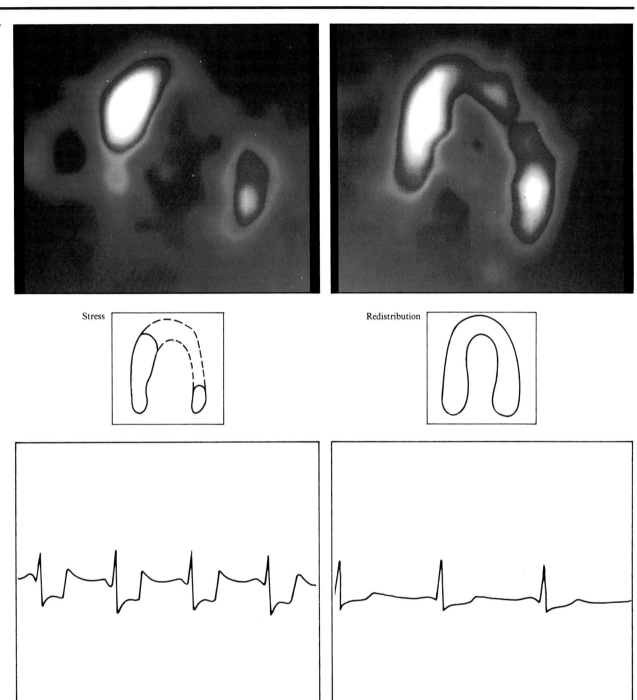

Stress (left) and redistribution (right) horizontal long axis tomograms (top) with ECG (bottom) showing reversible ischaemia of the lateral wall and basal septum. In this case, the abnormality was produced by intravenous infusion of dipyridamole and no exercise was necessary.

38 Normal left anterior oblique end diastolic image from an equilibrium radionuclide ventriculogram.

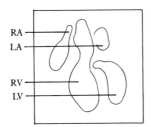

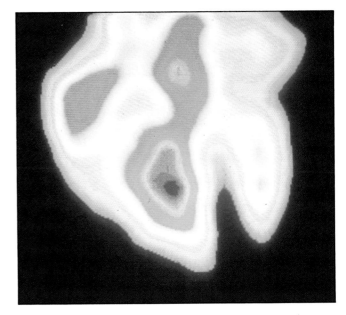

39 Normal amplitude image showing high amplitude of all parts of the left ventricle.

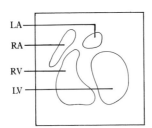

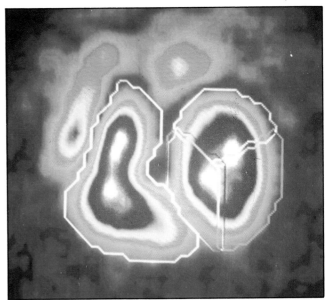

40 Normal phase image showing synchronous contraction of all parts of both ventricles in green. The atria and great vessels are 180° out of phase and are seen in red.

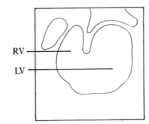

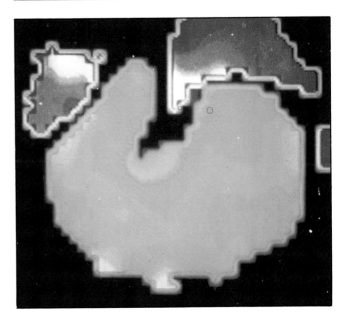

41

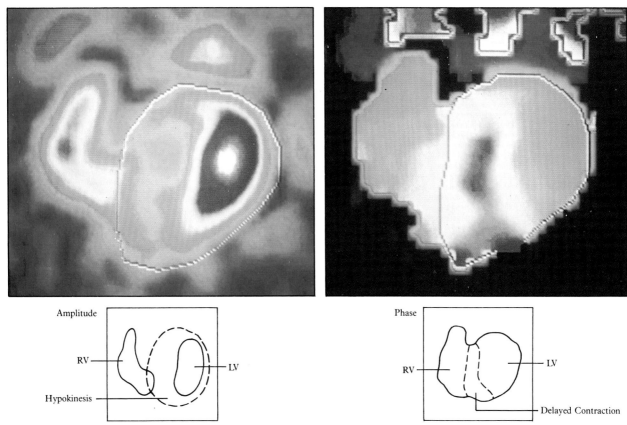

Amplitude (left) and phase (right) images in anteroseptal infarction. There are reduced values of amplitude and high phase in the region of the septum. This indicates hypokinesis and delayed contraction.

42

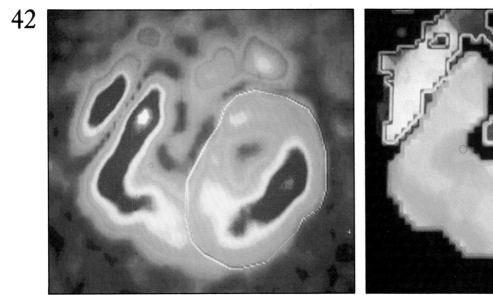
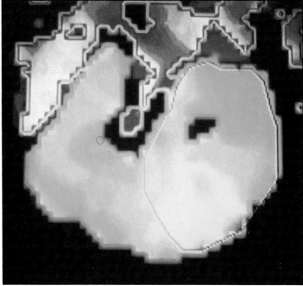
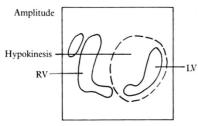
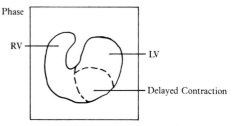

Amplitude (left) and phase (right) images in inferior infarction. The central amplitude defect and the delayed apical contraction are typical.

43 Phase image in left ventricular aneurysm showing apical dyskinesis (red).

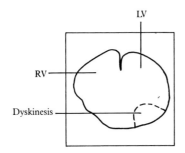

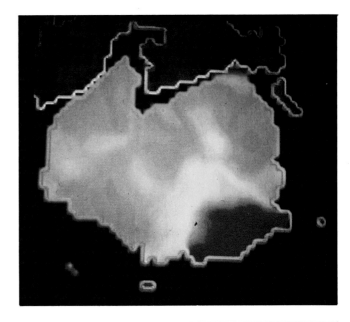

44

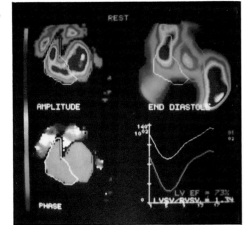

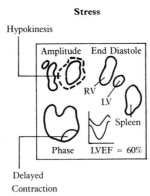

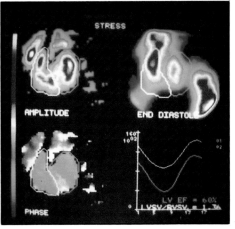

Rest (left) and stress (right) radionuclide ventriculograms with phase and amplitude images in a patient with coronary artery disease. The LVEF is normal at rest (73%) with normal regional wall motion shown on the amplitude and phase images. During stress, the LVEF falls (60%) and the amplitude and phase images show septal hypokinesis with delayed contraction.

45 Rest (left) and stress (right) amplitude and phase images. Regional wall motion is normal at rest, but delayed apical contraction develops during stress.

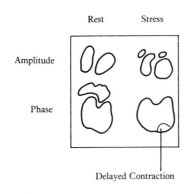

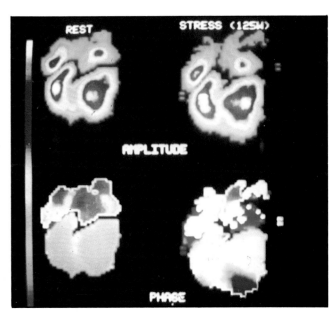

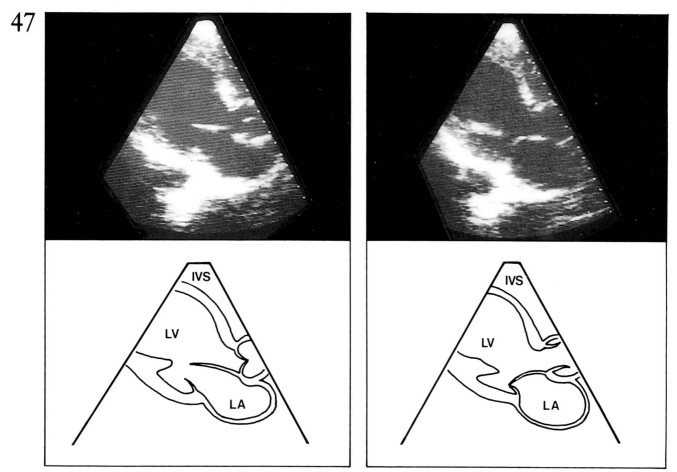

46 M-mode echocardiogram of the mitral valve (left) and left ventricle (right) in a patient with severe generalized left ventricular dysfunction due to coronary artery disease.

47 2-D echocardiographic parasternal long axis views in diastole (left) and systole (right) showing the thinning, anterior bulging and lack of movement of the septum following myocardial infarction.

48

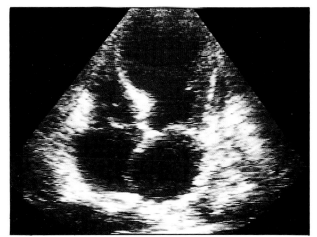 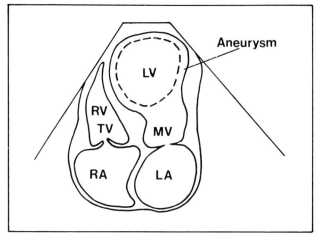

2-D echocardiographic apical four-chamber view of a large aneurysm.

49

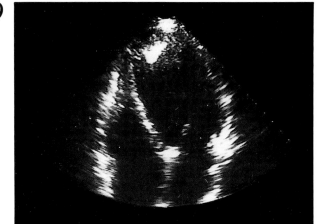 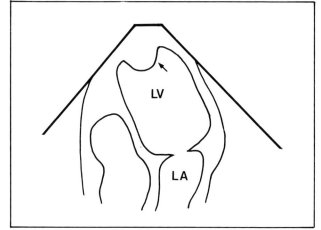

2-D echocardiographic apical four-chamber view of thrombus (arrow) in a patient with an old apical myocardial infarction.

50

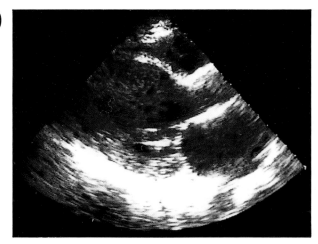 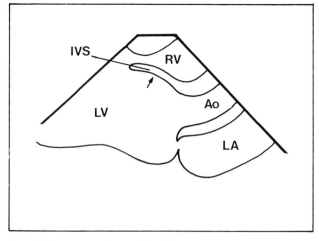

2-D echocardiographic systolic long axis view showing thinning of the septum (arrow) bulging into the right ventricle.

51

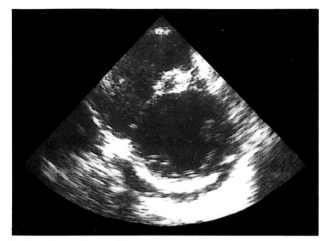
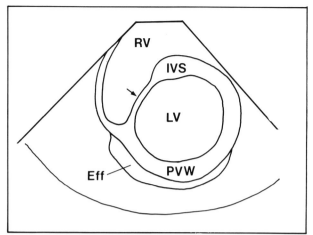

2-D echocardiographic systolic short axis view at level of papillary muscles in a patient with septal infarction. There is thinning of the septum (arrow) in relation to the anterior wall, and there is a pericardial effusion.

52

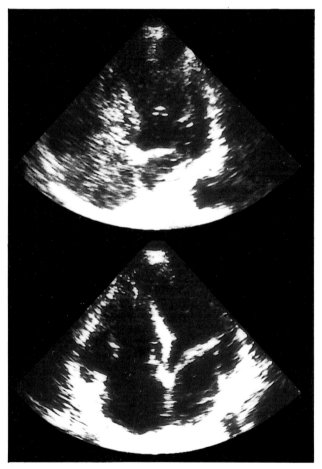
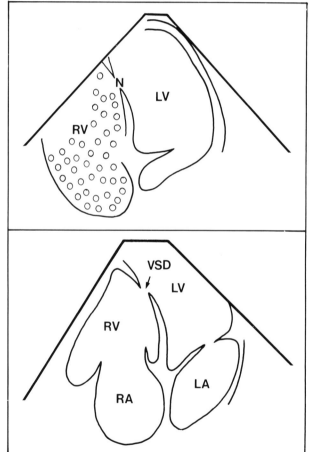

2-D echocardiographic four-chamber view in a patient with apico-septal ventricular septal defect after myocardial infarction. Above is a contrast injection into the right atrium and passing into the right ventricle. A negative contrast effect is seen in the right ventricle (N). Below is a non-contrast study in the same patient showing the ventricular septal defect (arrow) and a large right ventricle.

53

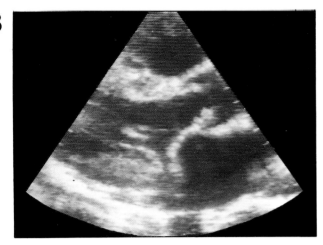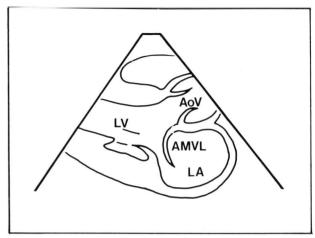

2-D echocardiographic parasternal long axis view showing 'flail' systolic motion of the anterior mitral valve leaflet into the left atrium.

ISCHAEMIC HEART DISEASE   Cardiac Catheterization & Angiography

54 Normal left coronary arteriogram in the right anterior oblique view.

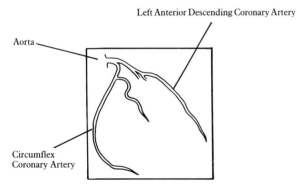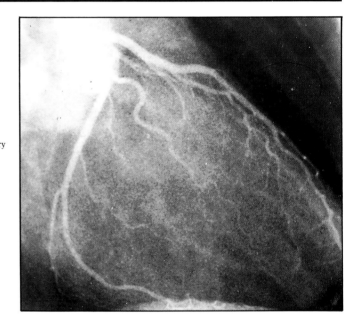

55 Angiogram in the left anterior oblique projection showing a normal left coronary artery.

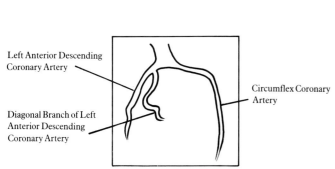

Left Anterior Descending Coronary Artery

Diagonal Branch of Left Anterior Descending Coronary Artery

Circumflex Coronary Artery

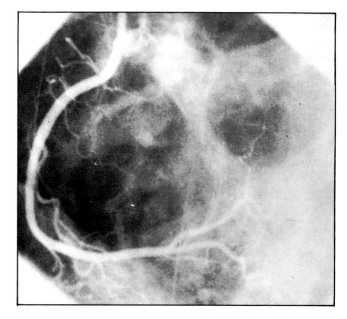

56 Angiogram in the left anterior oblique projection showing a normal right coronary artery.

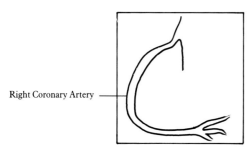

Right Coronary Artery

57 Angiogram showing atherosclerotic narrowing of the left anterior descending coronary artery (arrow).

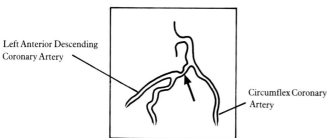

Left Anterior Descending Coronary Artery

Circumflex Coronary Artery

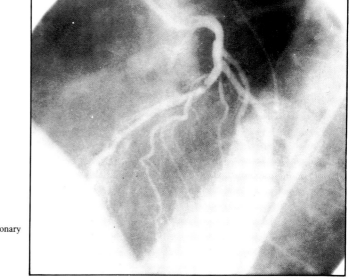

58 Angiogram showing atherosclerotic narrowing (arrow) of the left anterior descending coronary artery.

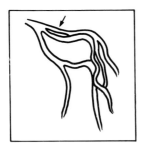

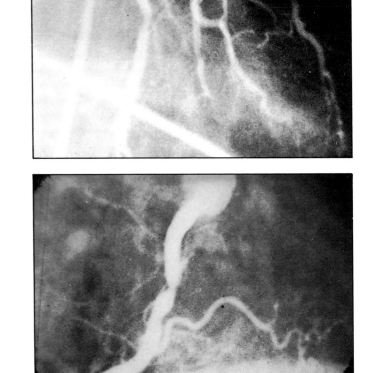

59 Right coronary angiogram viewed in the right anterior oblique projection showing obvious narrowing.

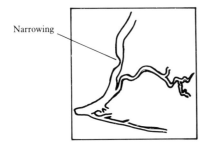

Narrowing

60 Right coronary angiogram viewed in the right anterior oblique projection showing diffuse disease of the artery with retrograde filling of the anterior descending coronary artery via septal collateral vessels.

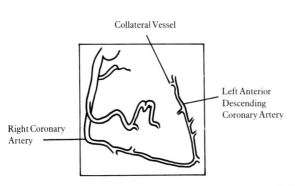

Collateral Vessel

Left Anterior
Descending
Coronary
Artery

Right Coronary
Artery

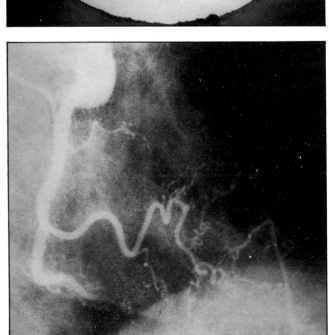

61

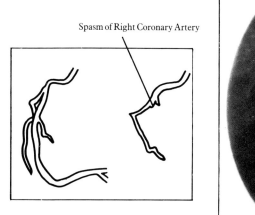

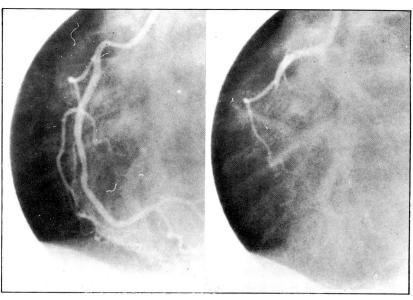

Coronary artery spasm. The angiogram on the left (left anterior oblique projection) shows normal blood flow in the right coronary artery. The angiogram on the right shows coronary artery spasm (arrow) completely occluding the right coronary artery.

62

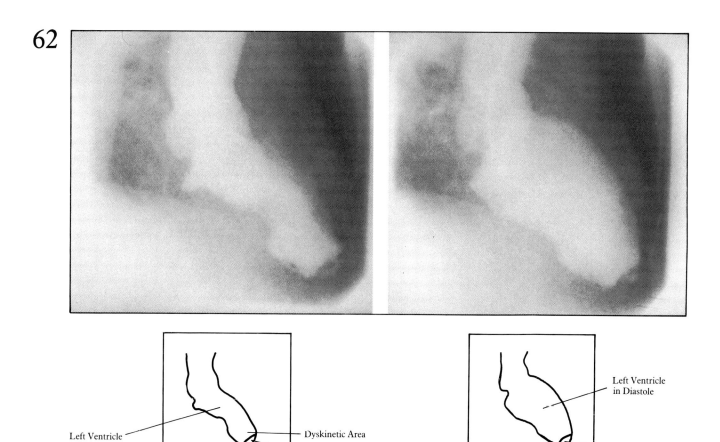

Left ventricular angiogram in the right anterior oblique projection. Systolic (left) and diastolic (right) frames reveal presence of apical dyskinesis and thrombus.

63

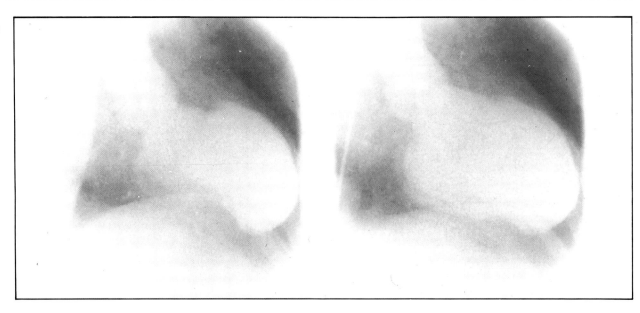

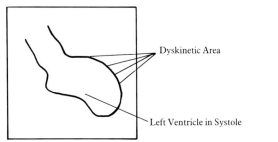

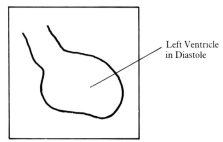

Left ventricular angiogram in the right anterior oblique projection with systolic (left) and diastolic (right) frames. It shows a large apical aneurysm with normal contraction of the remainder of the ventricle.

64

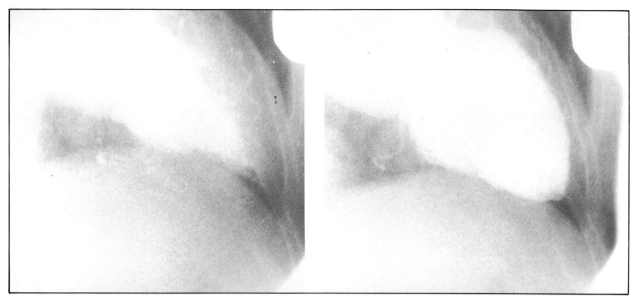

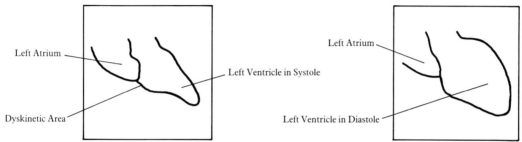

Left ventricular angiogram in the right anterior oblique projection with systolic (left) and diastolic (right) frames. It shows reduced contraction of the inferior wall of the left ventricle and dense opacification of the left atrium due to mitral regurgitation.

65 Left ventricular angiogram in the left anterior oblique projection showing a shunt from the left ventricle into the right ventricle due to rupture of the muscular septum.

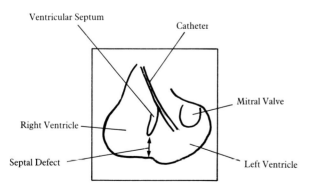

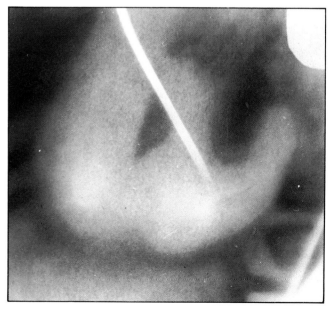

Chapter 2.

Heart Failure

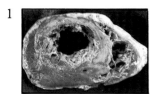

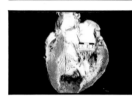

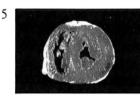

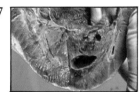

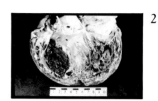

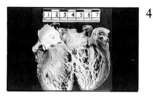

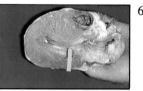

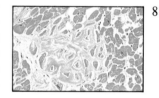

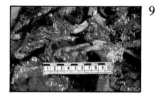

Pathology

The clinical syndrome of heart failure consists of breathlessness, evidence of poor tissue perfusion (fatigue, oliguria, drowsiness) and the consequences of stimulation of the sympathetic and renin-angiotensin-aldosterone systems (tachycardia, peripheral vasoconstriction, salt and water retention). The clinical features of heart failure may be caused by impairment of myocardial function or a structural abnormality. Investigation of the patient is necessary in order to determine the cardiac abnormality which has given rise to the clinical syndrome of heart failure.

The commonest pathological abnormality of the heart which gives rise to the clinical syndrome of heart failure is disease of the myocardium. Other causes such as valvular heart disease, congenital heart disease and pericardial disease will not be discussed in this text. In ischaemic heart disease (acute myocardial infarction [1] and chronic ischaemic myocardial damage [2] including left ventricular aneurysm [3]) and dilated cardiomyopathy [4], left ventricular dysfunction may be both systolic and diastolic. Myocardial dysfunction is predominantly diastolic in hypertensive heart disease, hypertrophic cardiomyopathy [5,6] and restrictive cardiomyopathy (e.g. endomyocardial fibrosis [7]). Other causes include specific heart-muscle disease such as alcohol related cardiomyopathy, myocarditis and thyroid disease which cause clinical syndromes indistinguishable from dilated cardiomyopathy. Amyloidosis [8] causes a syndrome similar to restrictive cardiomyopathy. High output states such as Paget's disease, arterio-venous fistula, anaemia and Beri-Beri can result in heart failure. Right ventricular dysfunction may accompany left ventricular dysfunction. Any cause of pulmonary hypertension, either acute (massive pulmonary embolism [9]) or chronic (chronic obstructive airways disease, primary pulmonary hypertension, chronic thrombo-embolic disease) may result in right ventricular myocardial dysfunction and clinical heart failure.

Symptoms

Acute heart failure presents with acute breathlessness and lack of perfusion of vital organs. Breathlessness is mainly caused by pulmonary congestion due to increased left ventricular filling pressure. Lying flat increases pulmonary venous pressure further and causes orthopnoea; this may progress to the development of frank pulmonary oedema causing attacks of breathlessness at night which wake the patient (paroxysmal nocturnal dyspnoea). Unlike acute heart failure the cause of breathlessness in chronic heart failure is less well understood, but is probably more related to reduced perfusion of the tissues than to pulmonary congestion. Occasionally, a non-productive cough may be the only symptom in heart failure. Pulmonary oedema is often incorrectly diagnosed as bronchitis. Fatigue in chronic heart failure is mainly due to the reduced cardiac reserve on exercise and inadequate blood flow to exercising muscles.

Acute heart failure may be precipitated by an alteration of cardiac rhythm in patients with pre-existing myocardial dysfunction, fresh damage to the myocardium (e.g. myocardial infarction or myocarditis), inappropriate alterations of therapy and rarely, infection or pulmonary infarction. Occasionally, no precipitating cause can be found.

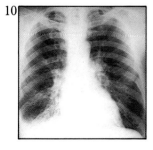

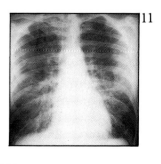

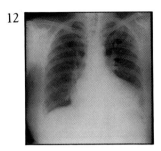

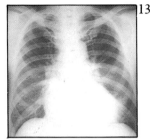

Patients with chronic heart failure may notice the development of fluid retention with swollen ankles and abdominal distention due to ascites or hepatic congestion. The patient with chronic heart failure may complain of nausea, vomiting and loss of weight due to gastrointestinal and hepatic congestion; such patients are frequently thought to have other abdominal pathology.

Acute right ventricular failure due to massive pulmonary embolism presents with circulatory collapse or acute breathlessness.

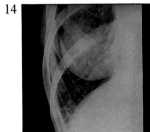

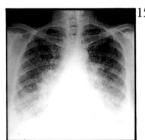

Signs

The physical signs may indicate whether heart failure is due to myocardial dysfunction or some other abnormality. Myocardial dysfunction renders the ventricles stiff and gives rise to a double apical impulse, a gallop rhythm (fourth and/or third heart sound) and secondary mitral or tricuspid regurgitation (pansystolic murmur); primary valvular abnormalities, congenital cardiac abnormalities or pericardial disease have distinctive clinical features.

Low cardiac output with stimulation of the sympathetic and renin-angiotensin-aldosterone systems will be associated with sinus tachycardia, peripheral vasoconstriction and fluid retention, causing a raised jugular venous pressure, pulmonary oedema, hepatic congestion, ascites and peripheral oedema. Renal, hepatic and cerebral impairment may also occur.

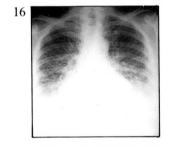

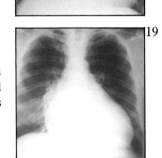

Investigations

Investigation of patients with clinical heart failure is essential in order to diagnose the cause. Valvular, congenital and pericardial disease may be detected but will not be discussed further in this section.

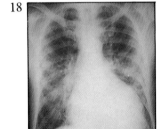

Radiology

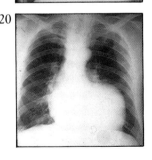

In patients presenting with 'acute' heart failure and breathlessness, the heart size may be normal [10,11] or enlarged. An enlarged heart implies pre-existing heart disease. The chest X-ray will show evidence of raised pulmonary venous pressure, such as dilatation of the upper zone pulmonary vessels, left atrial enlargement [12], Kerley B-lines (short horizontal lines in the peripheral lung fields [13,14]) and occasionally, unilateral or bilateral pleural effusions [15]; these findings correlate well with the elevation of left ventricular filling pressure and left atrial pressure and the consequent high pulmonary capillary wedge pressure. Pulmonary oedema is usually bilateral [16] but, occasionally, may be unilateral [17]. In 'chronic' heart failure the heart is usually enlarged and there may [18] or may not [19] be radiological features associated with raised pulmonary venous pressure. Characteristic radiological abnormalities are seen in acute pulmonary embolism, cor pulmonale, primary pulmonary hypertension and chronic thromboembolic disease. Features suggestive of a left ventricular aneurysm may also be seen [20].

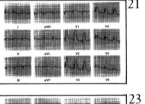

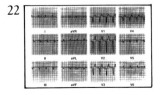

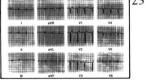

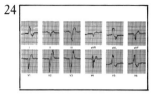

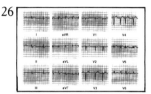

Electrocardiography

A normal ECG should alert the clinician to the possibility that the diagnosis of myocardial failure is incorrect. The ECG may show acute [21] or old [22] myocardial infarction, or evidence of left ventricular aneurysm [23]. Common abnormalities associated with chronic left ventricular dysfunction include left atrial configuration of the 'P' waves, left bundle branch block [24] or only ST/T abnormalities [25]. Patients with heart failure due to myocardial disease often have rhythm abnormalities which may be seen on the routine ECG [26,27] or may be detected only during 24 hour ambulatory monitoring [28]. Right ventricular dysfunction may be associated with right axis deviation and right bundle branch block or evidence of right ventricular hypertrophy.

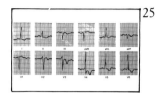

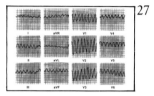

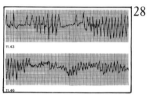

Echocardiography

The echocardiographic features will reflect the underlying cardiac abnormality. In patients with ischaemic heart disease, 2-dimensional echocardiography will show an increase in left ventricular dimensions and reduction in wall motion which may be either regional [29,30] or generalized [31]. Systolic wall thinning and/or dyskinesia are readily apparent from inspection of the systolic and diastolic images. A localized left ventricular aneurysm may be detected by 2-dimensional echocardiography [32] and thrombus within an abnormal ventricle may sometimes be seen [33]. In patients with dilated cardiomyopathy not due to ischaemic heart disease, the left ventricular dimensions are again increased and amplitude of wall motion is reduced globally [34]. Slight enlargement of the left atrium, due to chronic elevation of the left ventricular filling pressure, is common.

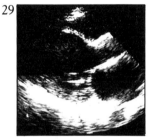

In hypertrophic cardiomyopathy there is marked left ventricular hypertrophy which may be concentric [35] or predominantly affecting the septum [36] or only the apex. The left ventricular cavity is small and may become obliterated in systole. Systolic anterior motion (SAM) of the anterior mitral valve leaflet may be seen [36] and there may be left atrial enlargement.

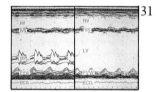

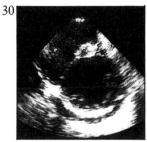

In restrictive cardiomyopathy, 2-dimensional echocardiography is helpful in the early diagnosis. Specific cavity changes such as apical and endocardial thickening can be demonstrated. Myocardial infiltration (e.g. endomyocardial fibrosis) gives a particular diagnostic reflection pattern on the grey scale and this can be further enhanced by amplitude process, colour-encoded tissue characterization techniques [37].

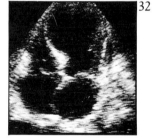

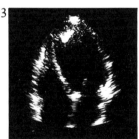

In patients with right heart failure due to pulmonary hypertension there may be evidence of paradoxical septal motion on M-mode echocardiography, and right ventricular hypertrophy and dilatation will be seen by 2-dimensional echocardiography.

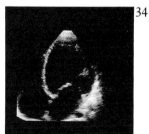

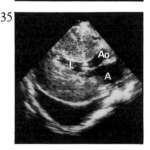

In patients with hypertensive heart disease, 2-dimensional echocardiography may show a hypertrophied but normally contracting left ventricle with diastolic dysfunction, but in more advanced disease, hypertrophy with a dilated and poorly contracting ventricle is seen.

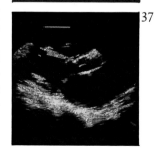

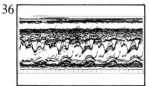

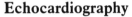

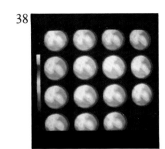

Nuclear Techniques

Nuclear techniques show functional information which complements the anatomical information provided by, for instance, coronary arteriography. An important nuclear cardiological procedure in patients with congestive heart failure is radionuclide ventriculography using technetium-99m to label the intracardiac blood pools. Imaging is either performed during the first passage of the bolus through the central circulation or when it has reached equilibrium [38,39]. Left ventricular volumes, ejection fraction and parameters of diastolic function such as filling rates can be measured [40]. Unfortunately, the ejection fraction is only an approximate indicator of ventricular performance and is poorly related to the severity of symptoms in congestive heart failure. Many variables in addition to ventricular function influence the ejection fraction, including ventricular preload and afterload. Regional wall motion can also be assessed and helpful methods of displaying both the extent and the timing of contraction are the Fourier amplitude and phase images [41-43]. Imaging during stress allows the response to exercise to be measured and a fall in LVEF and/or new regional wall motion abnormalities are suggestive of exercise induced ischaemia.

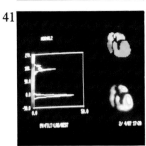

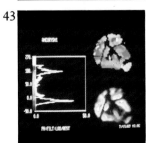

Regional myocardial perfusion abnormalities causing heart failure can be assessed by thallium-201 scintigraphy. It is possible to define normally perfused [44], reversibly ischaemic [45], and infarcted myocardium [46] and to assess the site and extent of abnormalities. Planar images have traditionally been used, but a significant advance has been the use of rotating gamma cameras to acquire images from many angles from which to reconstruct emission tomograms. The three dimensional view of myocardial perfusion provided by tomographic imaging greatly increases the accuracy of assessment and hence the clinical value of the technique. A further development that has increased the scope of the technique is the use of intravenous dipyridamole, a coronary arterial dilator, to induce abnormalities of thallium uptake in patients with coronary artery disease without the need for dynamic exercise [47].

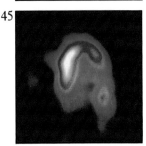

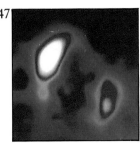

Positron emission tomography allows the imaging of radionuclides such as oxygen-15, nitrogen-13, fluorine-18, and carbon-11. Myocardial perfusion can be assessed quantitatively and myocardial metabolism can also be assessed with radio-pharmaceuticals such as flourine-18 deoxyglucose (FDG). In patients with congestive heart failure, regions with reduced perfusion but preserved metabolism (a change from fatty acid uptake to glucose uptake) have been termed 'hibernating myocardium'. Function returns in such areas following revascularization and so positron emission tomography is likely to gain increasing importance in the assessment of patients with ischaemic heart failure.

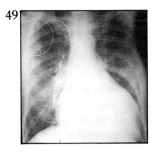

Cardiac Catheterization and Angiography

Bedside monitoring of right heart, haemodynamic variables can be useful in the management of patients with acute heart failure. A balloon-tipped thermodilution catheter [48] positioned with its tip in the pulmonary artery [49] allows accurate measurement of

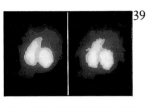

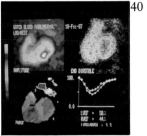

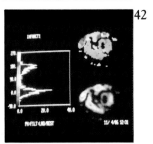

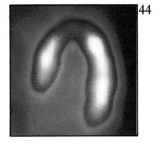

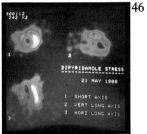

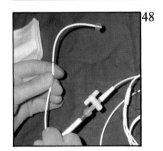

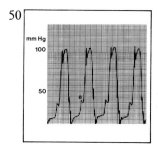

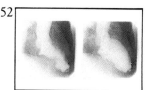

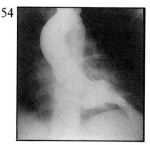

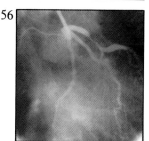

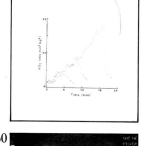

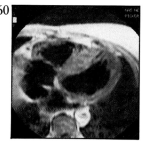

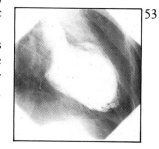

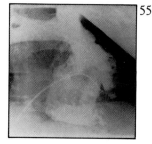

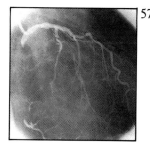

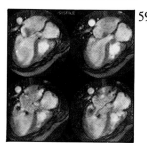

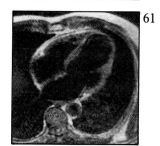

pulmonary artery and wedge pressure and cardiac output, facilitating accurate diagnosis.

In heart failure due to left ventricular disease, the left ventricular end-diastolic pressure is usually elevated, often with a prominent 'a' wave [50]. In hypertrophic cardiomyopathy, intracavity recordings may reveal left ventricular mid-cavity obstruction; restrictive cardiomyopathy causes characteristic haemodynamic abnormalities [51].

Left ventricular angiography is often unnecessary in patients with heart failure as non-invasive techniques will have defined the nature and degree of dysfunction. Localized hypokinesis [52] or left ventricular aneurysm may be seen following myocardial infarction. Alternatively, the left ventricle may be globally hypokinetic in generalized ischaemic heart disease or dilated cardiomyopathy [53]. Gross hypertrophy and systolic cavity obliteration is seen in hypertrophic cardiomyopathy [54]. Cavity obliteration and atrioventricular valvar regurgitation is also seen in restrictive cardiomyopathy [55].

Coronary arteriography is performed to demonstrate whether heart failure is due to coronary artery disease and, if so, to assess the possibilities of treatment. Localized stenoses [56] or, more often, widespread coronary disease may be found [57] even in the absence of a history of myocardial infarction or angina.

Exercise Testing

All the investigations referred to above assess the type and degree of left ventricular dysfunction rather than the clinical state of the patient. Exercise testing proves an objective measure of functional impairment in heart failure. Maximal or submaximal tests on a treadmill or bicycle ergometer, with measurement of exercise time or oxygen consumption [58] can be useful in the diagnosis and follow up of symptomatic patients.

Magnetic Resonance Imaging

Magnetic resonance images are maps of the radio signals emitted by the photons within the body (mainly those in water and fat) under the influence of a powerful magnetic field. They reveal cardiac anatomy noninvasively and without the injection of contrast media. Accurate measurements of ventricular volumes [59], wall thickness [60a & 60b] and wall motion [61] can be made, and filling defects such as thrombus are readily detected. The images can be acquired as cine loops to demonstrate moving anatomy, and the turbulence of valvular disease and intracardiac shunting can be encoded in the phase of the magnetic resonance signal. Cine velocity mapping holds great potential for the assessment of vascular disease.

In patients with heart failure, the main application of magnetic resonance imaging is in the accurate measurement and follow up of ventricular function, the detection of thrombus, and the assessment of associated lesions such as mitral regurgitation.

1 Transverse slice (fresh) of the ventricles. A recent (four-day-old) full-thickness myocardial infarction is present in the anterior wall of the left ventricle which extends into the interventricular septum.

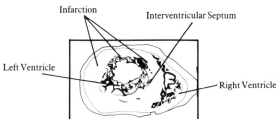

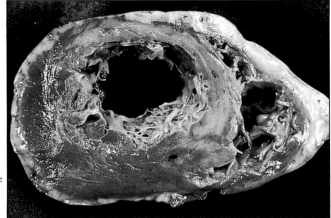

2 Widespread ischaemic scarring of the myocardium producing a dilated thin-walled ventricle. A thrombus has formed in one area in relation to the aneurysmal bulge of the ventricular wall.

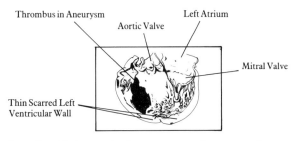

3 Localized left ventricular aneurysm due to previous myocardial infarction. The aneurysm does not contain more than a fine deposit of thrombus and has a larger central cavity opening into the ventricle.

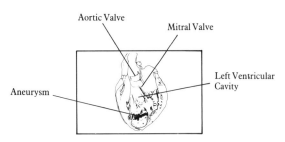

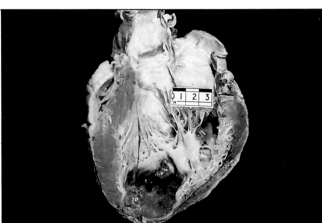

4 Dilated cardiomyopathy: the opened left ventricle has a large cavity and thin wall.

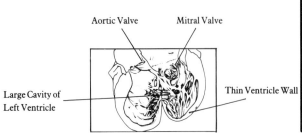

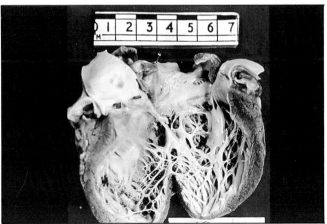

5 Transverse section through heart in hypertrophic cardiomyopathy showing concentric left ventricular hypertrophy.

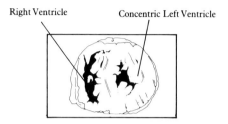

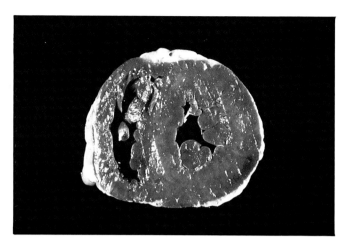

6 The left ventricle from a patient with hypertrophic cardiomyopathy showing a small cavity with very thick wall. The septal region is asymmetrically thickened being at least twice as thick as the parietal wall. The septum bulges into the outflow tract of the left ventricle and impinges onto the anterior cusp of the mitral valve (arrow).

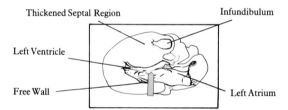

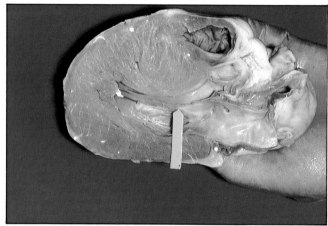

7 Section through the left ventricle in endomyocardial fibrosis. There is marked left ventricular apical obliteration with endocardial thickening and super-added thrombus.

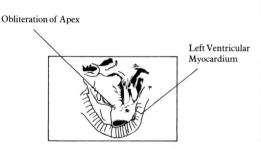

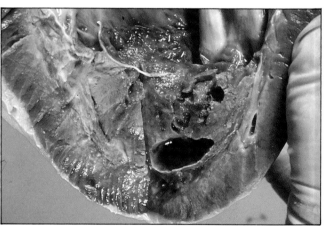

8 Amyloid deposition in the myocardium. In haematoxylin and eosin stained histological sections amyloid is a pale pink homogeneous material. Amyloid (arrows) is laid down between myocardial cells and ultimately completely surrounds them leaving a lattice of amyloid within which a few residual muscle cells are embedded, staining a deeper pink colour.

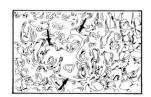

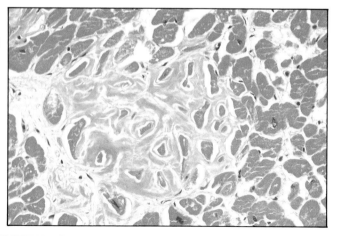

9   Large saddle embolus is seen astride both right and left pulmonary arteries.

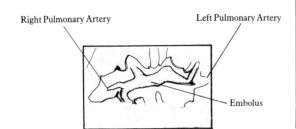

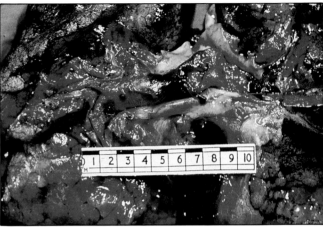

10   Chest radiograph showing a normal sized heart with upper lobe venous distention and a small right pleural effusion, due to recent myocardial infarction.

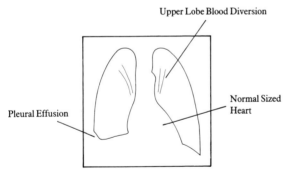

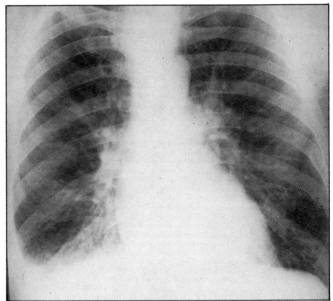

11 Chest radiograph showing a normal sized heart with pulmonary oedema.

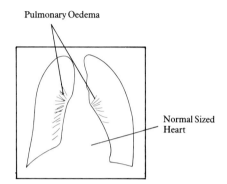
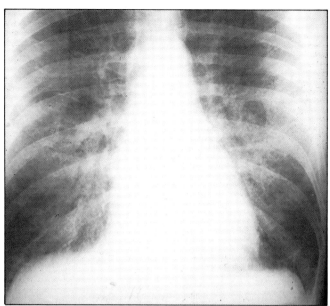

12 Chest radiograph showing large heart and left atrium with pulmonary venous hypertension.

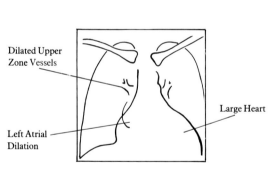
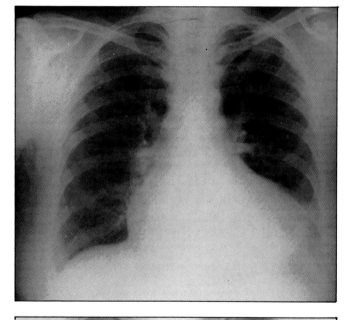

13 Chest radiograph showing cardiomegaly, upper lobe pulmonary venous distention and Kerley B-lines.

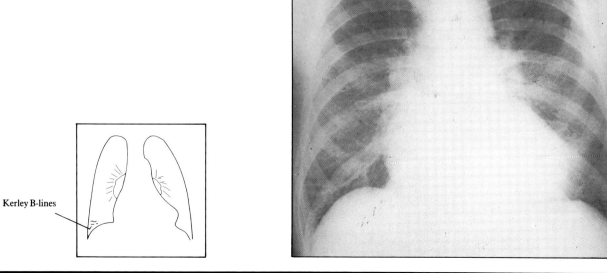

14 Detail from chest radiograph showing septal lines and pleural effusion.

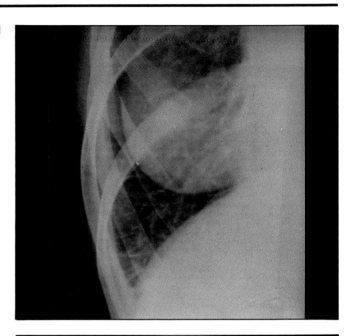

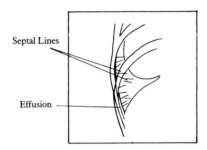

15 Chest radiograph showing pulmonary oedema and bilateral pleural effusions following acute myocardial infarction.

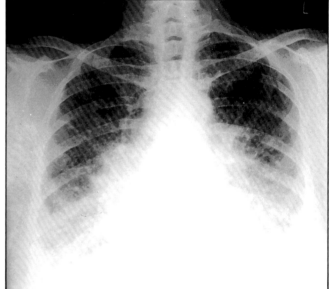

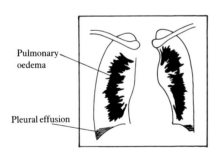

16 Chest radiograph in acute heart failure due to acute myocardial infarction. There is gross pulmonary oedema.

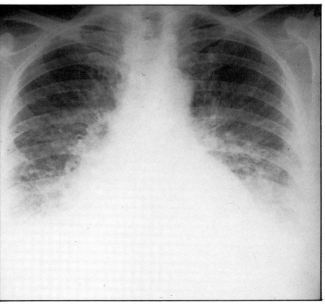

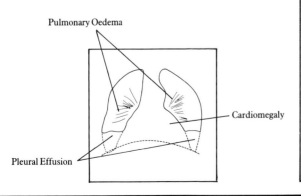

17 Chest radiograph showing cardiomegaly and pulmonary oedema of the right lung only.

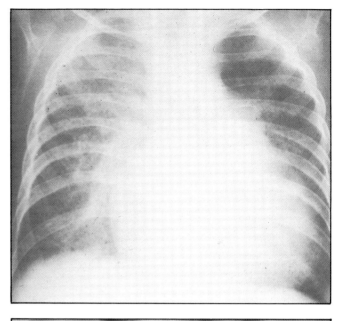

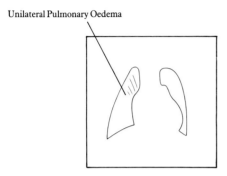

18 Chest radiograph showing cardiomegaly with features of raised pulmonary venous pressure (enlarged veins and upper zone blood diversion).

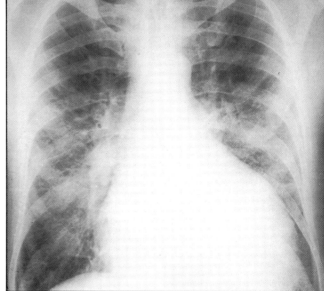

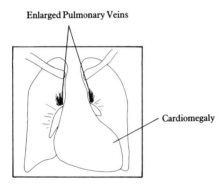

19 Chest radiograph showing an enlarged heart without upper zone blood diversion.

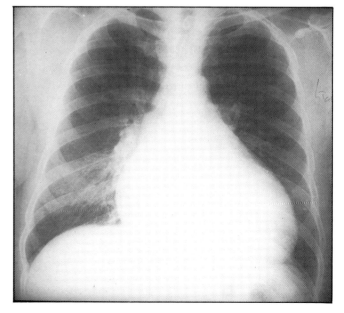

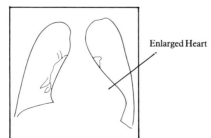

20   Chest radiograph showing a bulge on the left heart border suggestive of a left ventricular aneurysm.

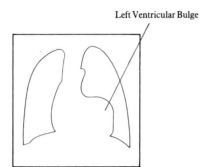

Left Ventricular Bulge

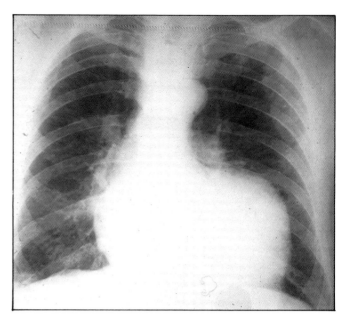

21

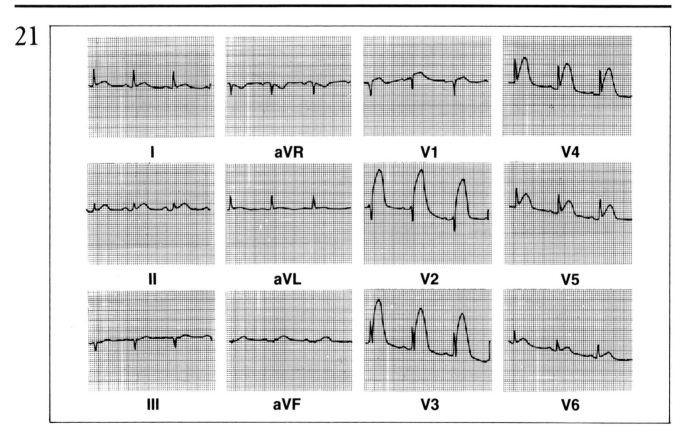

I   aVR   V1   V4

II   aVL   V2   V5

III   aVF   V3   V6

Electrocardiogram showing the very early changes of anterior myocardial infarction (30 min after onset of pain). There is ST elevation in leads I, II, and across all the V leads, but no Q wave development yet.

22

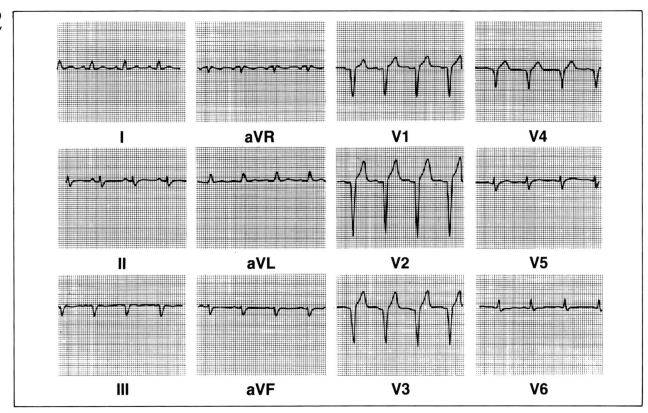

Electrocardiogram of a patient with chronic ischaemic heart disease, showing old anterior infarction, with Q waves in V_{1-4} and poor R wave progression in V_{5-6}.

23

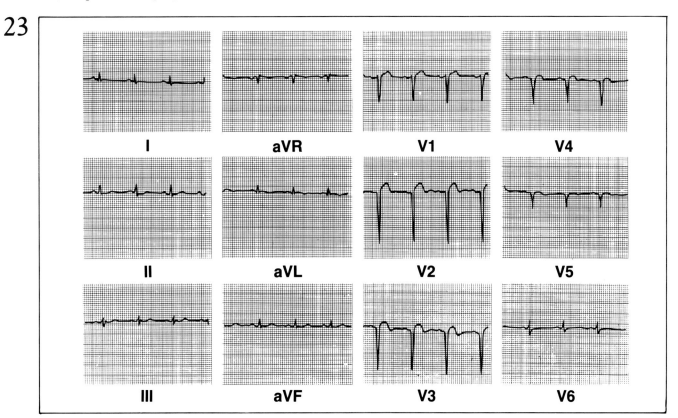

Electrocardiogram in a patient with left ventricular aneurysm, showing Q waves and persistent ST elevation in the anterior chest leads, six months after myocardial infarction.

24

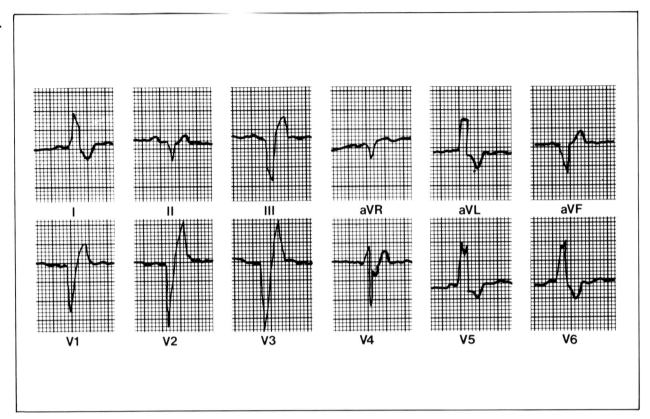

Electrocardiogram in a patient with dilated cardiomyopathy showing left bundle branch block.

25

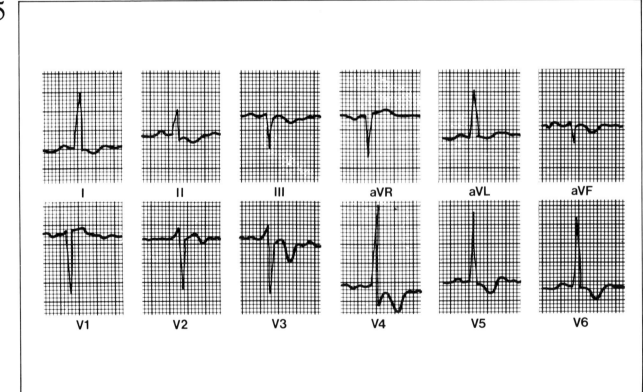

Electrocardiogram in a patient with dilated cardiomyopathy showing non-specific ST/T abnormalities.

26

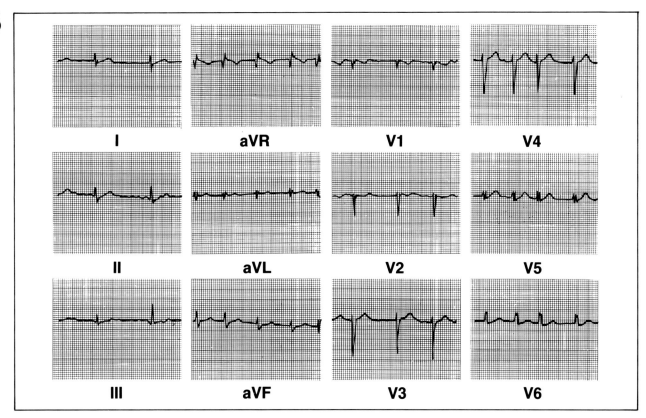

Electrocardiogram of a patient with dilated cardiomyopathy, showing atrial fibrillation, poor R wave progression in the chest leads, and partial left bundle branch block, but no Q waves.

27

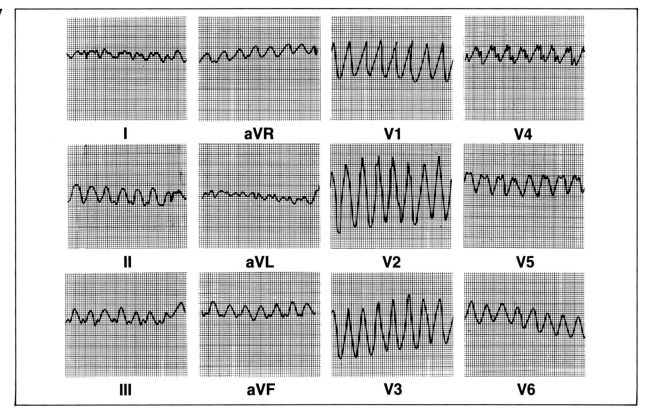

Electrocardiogram recorded from a patient with dilated cardiomyopathy, taken when he complained of dizziness. The 12 lead ECG shows ventricular tachycardia.

28

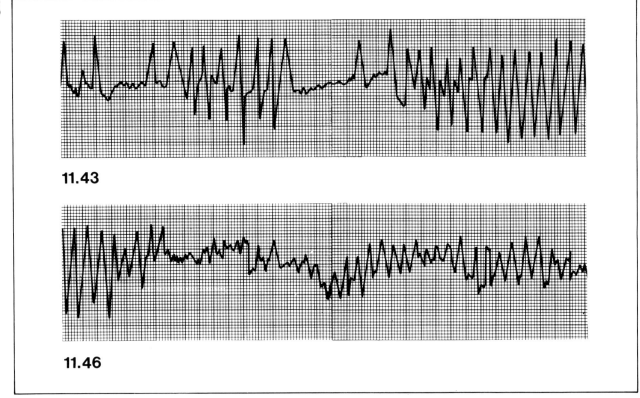

11.43

11.46

Ambulatory ECG recording from a patient with heart failure. On returning home with the recorder at 11.35, the patient sat down to drink a cup of coffee. At 11.43 he developed ventricular tachycardia and collapsed. At 11.46 ventricular fibrillation developed and the patient died.

29

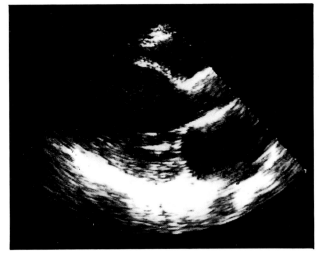 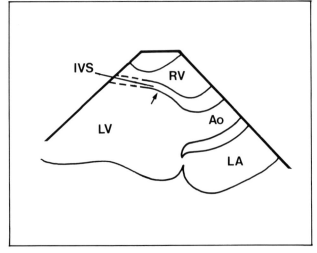

2-D echocardiographic systolic long axis view in a patient with septal infarction showing thinning of the septum (arrow) bulging into the right ventricle.

30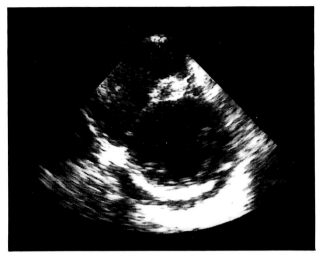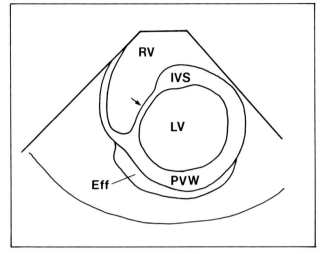

2-D echocardiographic systolic short axis view at level of papillary muscles in a patient with septal infarction. There is thinning of the septum (arrow) in relation to the anterior wall, and there is a pericardial effusion.

31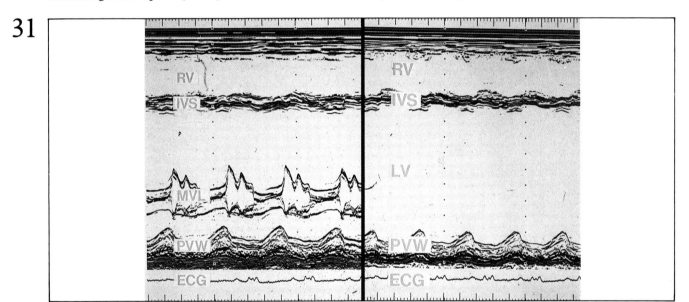

M-mode echocardiogram of the mitral valve (left) and left ventricle (right) in a patient with severe generalized left ventricular dysfunction due to coronary artery disease.

32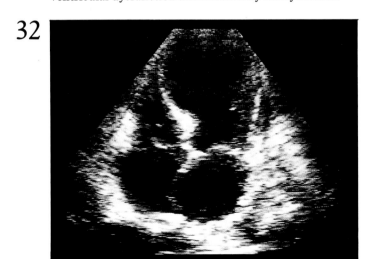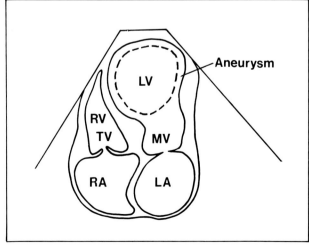

2-D echocardiographic apical four-chamber view showing a large left ventricular aneurysm.

33
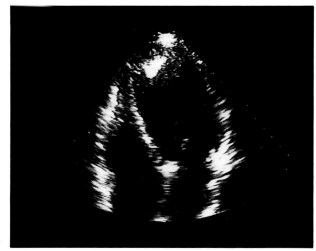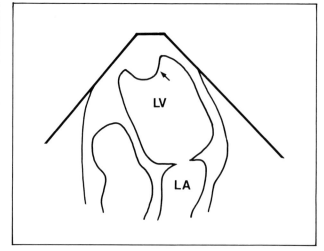

2-D echocardiographic apical four-chamber view showing apical thrombus (arrow) in a patient with an old apical myocardial infarction.

34
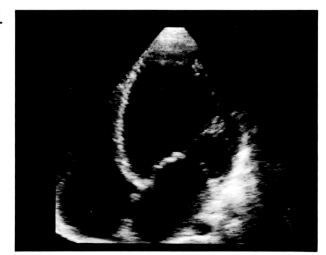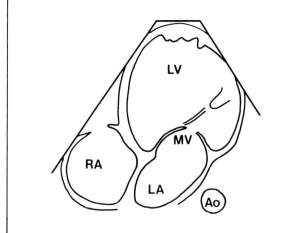

2-D echocardiographic apical four-chamber view showing left ventricular dilatation in dilated cardiomyopathy. Note the thin-walled globular left ventricle. The irregularities in the apex may be due to mural thrombus.

35
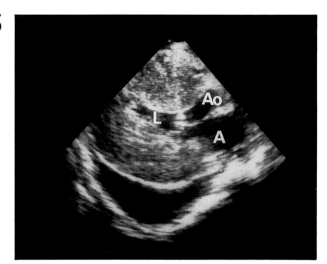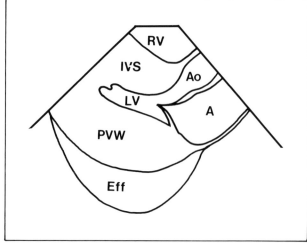

2-D echocardiographic parasternal long axis systolic view in hypertrophic cardiomyopathy with gross symmetrical hypertrophy of the left ventricle and slit-like cavity. Note additional pericardial effusion.

36
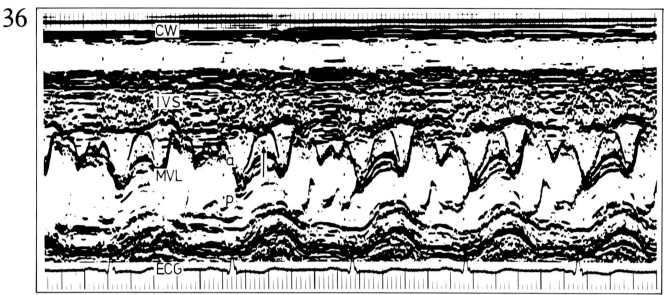

M-mode echocardiogram of hypertrophic cardiomyopathy with left ventricular outflow obstruction. The echocardiogram shows systolic anterior movement of the anterior leaflet (arrowed) which also strikes the septum at the onset of diastole.

37
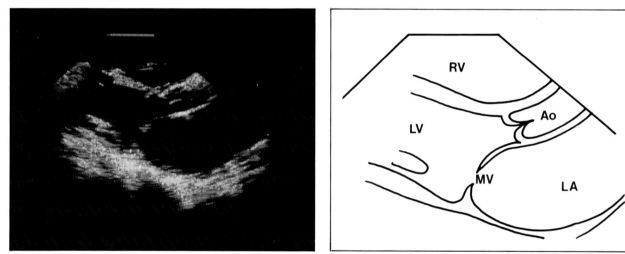

2-D echocardiographic amplitude processed colour-encoded long axis parasternal view in endomyocardial fibrosis showing increased echo density and endocardial thickening on the posterior left ventricular wall, thickening and tethering of the posterior mitral valve leaflet and left atrial dilatation.

38 Gated blood pool scan in a normal subject : 16 frames have been acquired (end systole at frame 4, end diastole at frame 1).

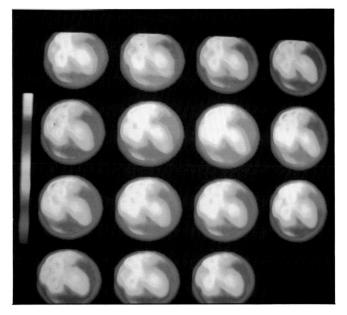

39 Gated blood pool scan in dilated cardiomyopathy showing little difference in the size of the ventricular cavities between end-diastole (left) and end-systole (right).

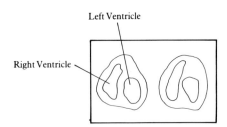

Left Ventricle

Right Ventricle

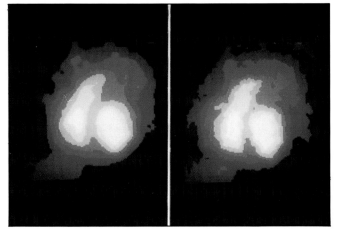

40 End-diastolic frames of equilibrium gated blood pool scans (top right) with regions of interest outlining the right and left ventricular cavities. By measuring the counts in these regions throughout the cardiac cycle, an accurate measure of the change in cavity volume can be made, to yield volume curves and calculated ejection fractions (EF) (bottom right);
a) Normal (LVEF 58%, RVEF 44%),
b) LV aneurysm (LVEF 23%, RVEF 24%),
c) Dilated cardiomyopathy (LVEF 10%, RVEF 11%).

(a)

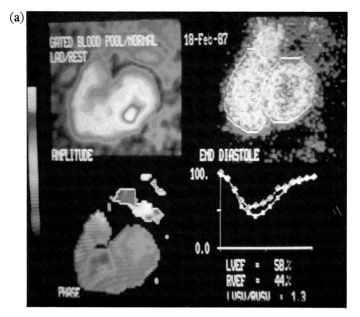

(b)

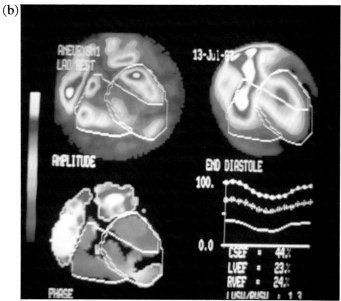

(c)

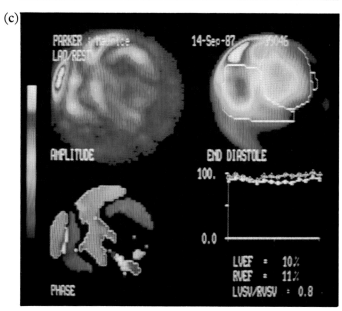

41 Parametric imaging. By constructing volume curves throughout the cardiac cycle from each pixel of a gated blood pool scan, the computer can generate colour-encoded images of amplitude of regional wall motion, and phase of wall motion. In this normal heart the amplitude image (bottom right) shows vigorous left ventricular contraction. The phase image (top right) shows both ventricles contract uniformly and in synchrony (coded blue), with the atria 180° out of phase (i.e. contract in diastole) (coded red), giving two sharp peaks at 0° and 180° on the phase histogram.

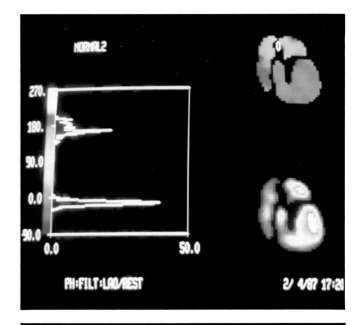

42 Parametric images following myocardial infarction. The amplitude image reveals poor amplitude of left ventricular wall motion. The phase image is fragmented, showing discoordinate ventricular contraction, giving poorly defined peaks on the phase histogram.

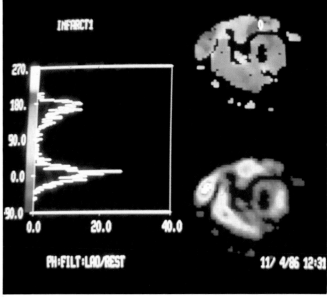

43 Parametric images from a patient with left ventricular aneurysm. The amplitude image shows reduced apical movement and the phase image shows clearly that motion of the apex is out of phase compared to the rest of the ventricle.

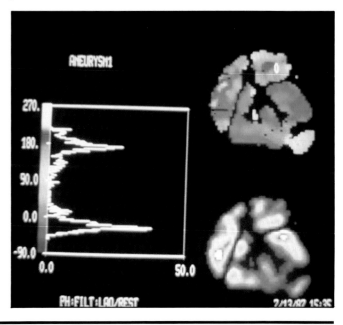

44 Normal thallium-201 myocardial perfusion emission tomograms in vertical and horizontal long axis and short axis planes. There is uniform uptake of thallium throughout the myocardium.

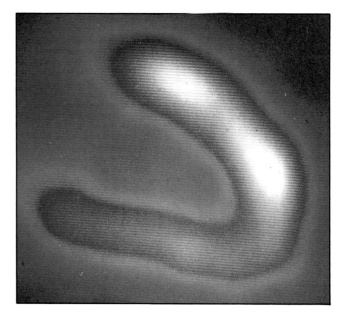

Vertical Long Axis

Anterior

Inferior

Apex

Horizontal Long Axis

Apex

Septum

Lateral

Short Axis

Anterior

Septum

Lateral

Inferior

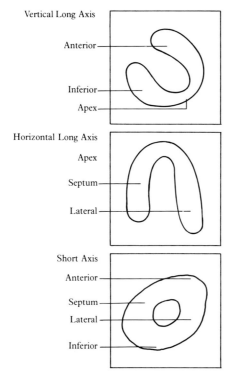

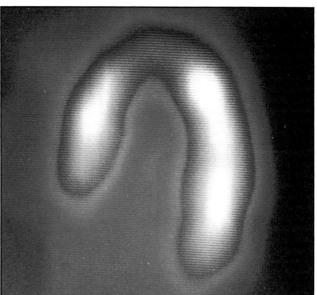

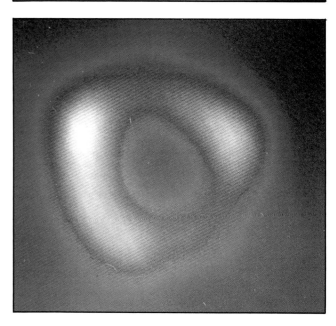

45 Stress and redistribution horizontal long axis
tomograms showing reversible lateral wall
ischaemia in a patient with left circumflex
coronary artery disease. The extent of ischaemia
is limited.

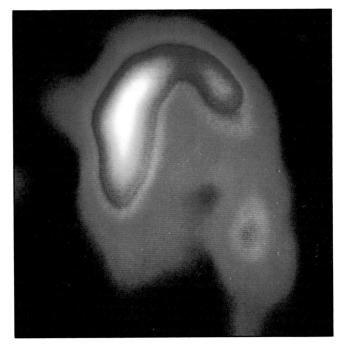

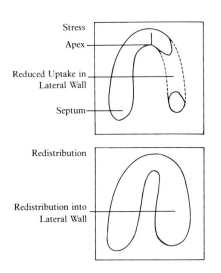

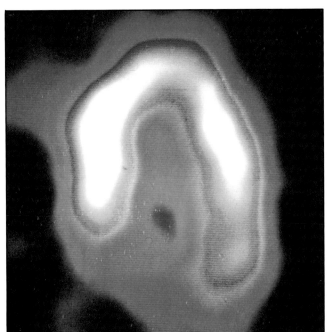

46 Stress and redistribution tomograms showing inferior infarction and reversible anteroseptal and apical ischaemia. The patient presented with congestive heart failure.

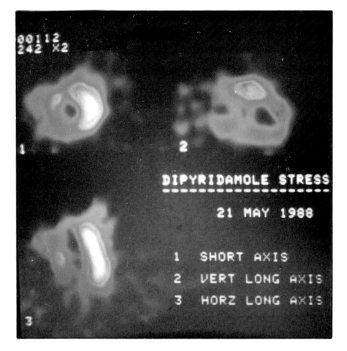

Stress

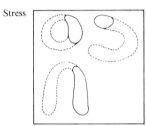

Redistribution

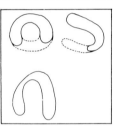

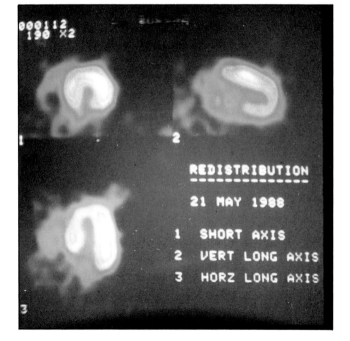

47

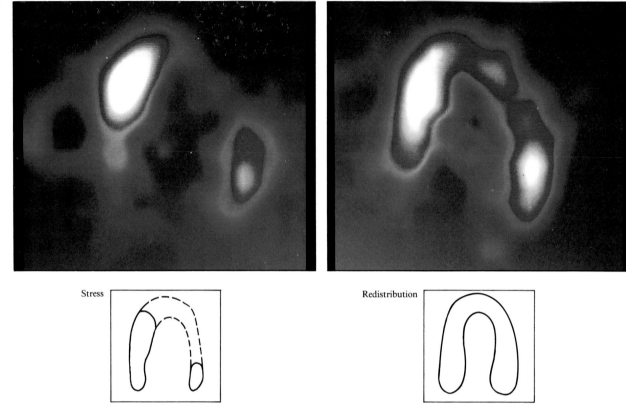

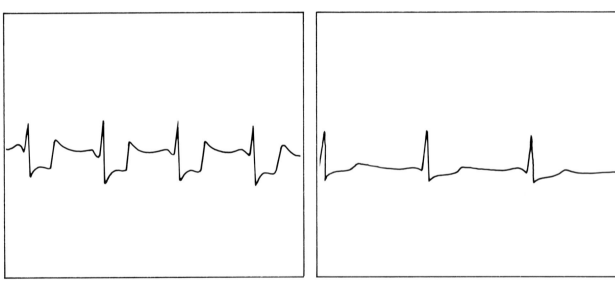

Stress and redistribution horizontal long axis tomograms with ECG showing reversible ischaemia of the lateral wall and basal septum. In this case, the abnormality was induced by intravenous infusion of dipyridamole and no exercise was necessary.

48 A balloon-tipped thermodilution catheter for right heart haemodynamic monitoring.

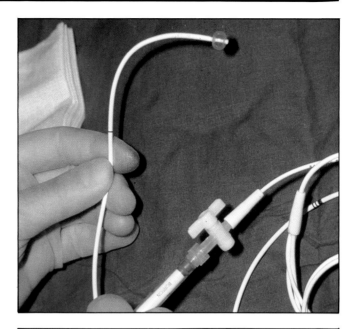

49 Chest radiograph showing a catheter inserted via the right subclavian vein, positioned with its tip in the right pulmonary artery for measurement of wedge pressure.

Balloon Tipped Catheter

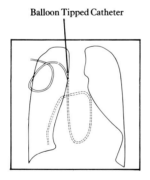

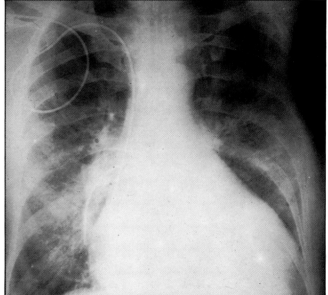

50 Pressure recording from the left ventricle in a patient with heart failure. The end-diastolic pressure is raised and there is a prominent 'a' wave.

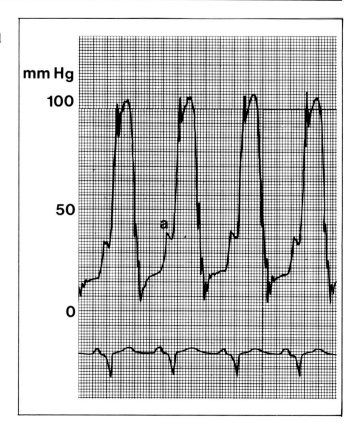

51 Pressure recordings taken from the right and left ventricles simultaneously in endomyocardial fibrosis showing the typical 'dip and plateau' and the elevated and different end diastolic pressure measurements.

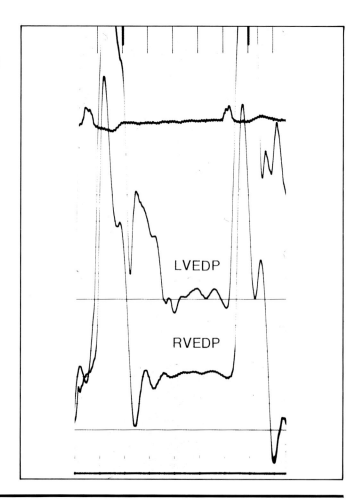

52

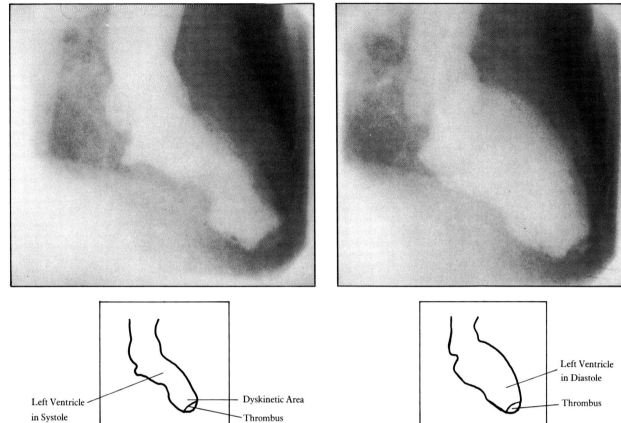

Left ventricular angiogram in the right anterior oblique projection. Systolic (left) and diastolic (right) frames reveal presence of apical dyskinesis and thrombus.

53

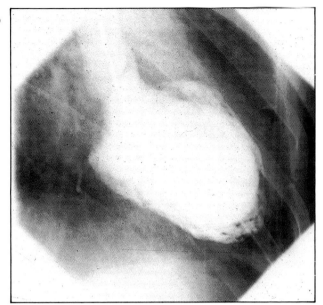
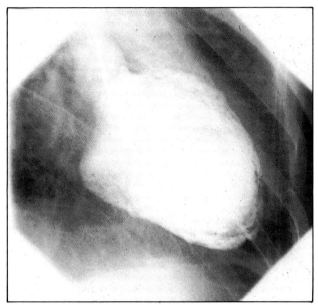

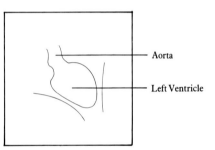
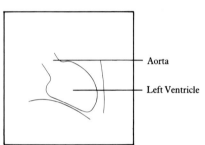

Left ventricular angiogram in the right anterior oblique projection with systolic (left) and diastolic (right) frames showing global hypokinesis and ventricular dilatation.

54 Left ventricular angiogram in hypertrophic cardiomyopathy showing in systole (antero-posterior projection) a small irregular cavity.

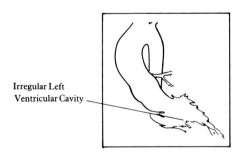
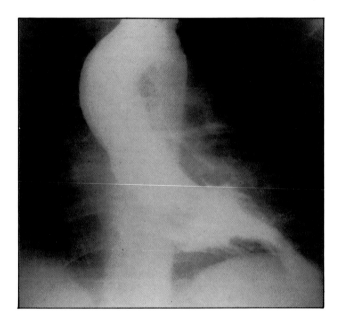

55 Right ventricular angiogram showing apical cavity obliteration and tricuspid regurgitation due to endomyocardial fibrosis.

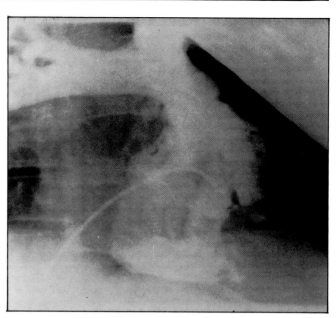

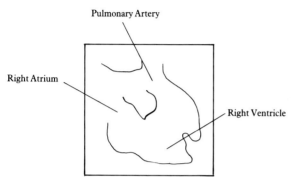

56 Coronary arteriogram (right anterior oblique projection) showing a long severe narrowing of the left anterior descending coronary artery.

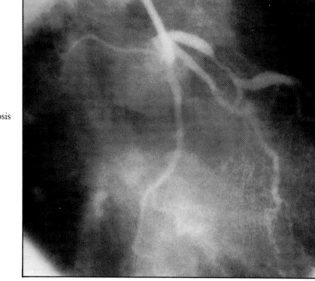

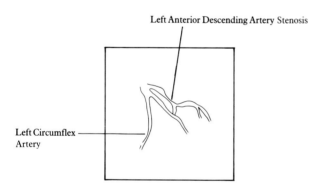

57 Coronary arteriogram (right anterior oblique projection) in three vessel coronary disease. The left coronary has been injected showing extensive disease, with retrograde filling of the right coronary artery.

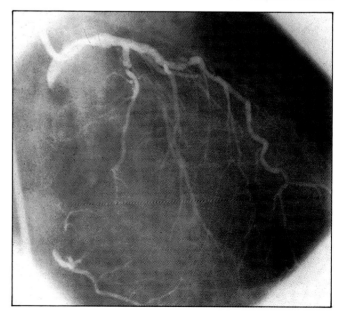

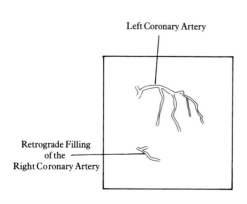

58 Oxygen consumption (VO_2) during symptom limited treadmill exercise and on recovery, in a normal subject (right), a patient with moderate heart failure (middle) and a patient with severe heart failure (left). At rest and during the first 5 minutes of exercise all three subjects have similar oxygen consumption, but peak VO_2 is progressively reduced with increasing heart failure.

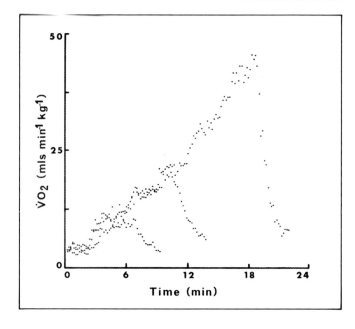

59 Magnetic resonance imaging in dilated cardiomyopathy. Four frames from a cine acquisition in the horizontal long axis plane using a field echo sequence where blood appears with high signal (white) except where there is turbulence. There is global left ventricular hypokinesia.

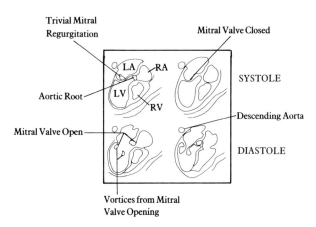

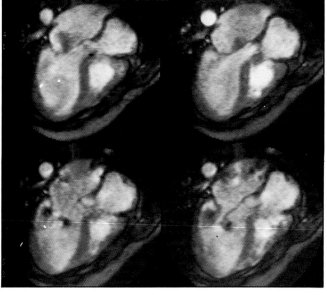

60 Magnetic resonance imaging in hypertrophic cardiomyopathy (HCM). Diastolic (a) and systolic (b) transverse sections showing asymmetric septal hypertrophy. The high signal from the septal myocardium is a consequence of altered relaxation times in the abnormal muscle.

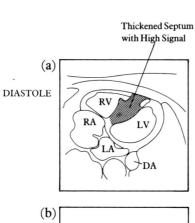

(a) DIASTOLE

Thickened Septum with High Signal

RV
RA
LV
LA
DA

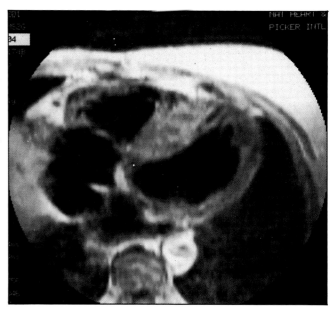

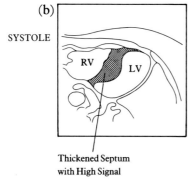

(b) SYSTOLE

RV
LV

Thickened Septum with High Signal

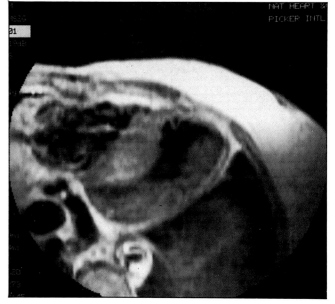

61

Magnetic resonance imaging in left ventricular aneurysm. Diastolic (left) and systolic (right) transverse sections in a patient with previous infarction and an apical left ventricular aneurysm. The basal myocardium contracts well whilst the apical myocardium is thin and dyskinetic.

Chapter 3.
Hypertension

HYPERTENSION

Prevalence

Hypertension is defined by selecting an arbitrary cut-off point for systolic and diastolic blood pressures. Since there is no natural dividing line, the proportion of hypertensive patients in any population depends upon the judgement of the observer [1]. The most widely used criterion is that chosen by the Expert Sub-Committee of the World Health Organisation i.e. 160/95 mmHg or above. Using this criterion the prevalence of hypertension ranges from about 3% in subjects below the age of 20 to over 40% of the male population in the older age groups. The overall prevalence on single readings lies between 15% and 20%. When repeated measurements are taken the observed blood pressure falls and therefore the observed prevalence of hypertension falls *pari passu*.

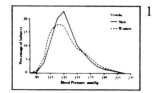

High blood pressure is a multifactorial condition in which both environmental and genetic factors play an important part. It is, for instance, more common in obese subjects, in those consuming large amounts of alcohol and in subjects with a strong family history of this condition. Hypertension is commonly classified according to its cause. Individuals in whom the only apparent factor is a genetic predisposition are regarded as having primary or essential hypertension, whilst individuals in whom a specific cause can be identified are regarded as having secondary hypertension. This subdivision, whilst convenient, suffers from the disadvantage that the overwhelming majority of hypertensive patients in the given population will have essential hypertension. The true prevalence of the two classes of hypertension is difficult to establish as most specialists in the area deal with highly selected populations usually biased towards secondary hypertension. However, it is unlikely that more than 5% of hypertensive population suffer from secondary hypertension. When evident causes such as obesity, alcohol and the contraceptive pill are excluded, the true prevalence of secondary hypertension is probably less than 1%.

Hypertension can also be classified into so called 'benign' or 'accelerated' (malignant) hypertension. Although this is a clinically useful subdivision, the term 'benign' is a misnomer as any chronic elevation of blood pressure carries an increased risk of strokes, heart attacks and peripheral vascular disease. In addition, the same patient may show evidence of both benign and accelerated hypertension at different times. Accelerated hypertension is best considered as a phase in either essential or secondary hypertension characterized by certain clinical and pathological features.

Pathology

Hypertension gives rise to changes throughout the arterial tree. Pathological changes may also occur in organs supplied by those vessels ('target organs'). In addition, some of the conditions which cause hypertension may give rise to pathological appearances in the relevant tissues. Such causes are shown in Table 1.

Table 1
Causes of Secondary Hypertension

Reno-vascular,	Renal Parenchymal,	Endocrine,
Pregnancy,	Medications,	Coarctation,
Neurological,	Dietetic (alcohol and obesity)	

Renal Hypertension

Diseases of the renal blood vessels may cause hypertension (renovascular hypertension) as may diseases of the kidney itself (renal parenchymal hypertension).

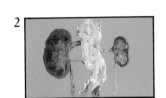

Renovascular hypertension is produced by unilateral or bilateral renal ischaemia [2,3]. The two commonest causes of this are atheroma of the renal arteries and fibromuscular dysplasia. The former causes discrete areas of narrowing associated with atheromatous plaques, most commonly situated at the mouth of the renal artery. The most common form of fibromuscular dysplasia gives rise to regular fibromuscular ridges separated by thin segments of the vessel wall. The cause is unknown but it usually occurs in a younger age group than atheroma and is more common in female patients and smokers.

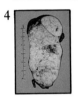

In addition to these intrinsic diseases of the renal artery, ischaemia may be produced by fibrous bands compressing the vessel or by tumours [4].

The three commonest forms of renal parenchymal disease giving rise to hypertension are chronic pyelonephritis [5], chronic glomerulonephritis and polycystic kidney. Hypertension may also be seen in less common diseases affecting the kidney such as scleroderma [6], polyarteritis nodosa, disseminated lupus erythematosus and analgesic nephropathy.

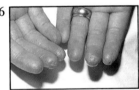

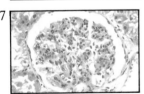

Hypertension is a common feature of acute glomerulonephritis and is seen in most patients with proliferative glomerulonephritis [7] at some stage in the course of their disease. It is less common in membranous glomerulonephritis [8] and not observed in minimal change nephropathy [9]. Macroscopically, in the acute stage of glomerulonephritis the kidneys may be swollen but as chronic glomerulonephritis proceeds they become shrunken. The more florid, proliferative glomerular changes are associated with more severe degrees of hypertension.

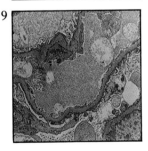

Endocrine Causes of Hypertension

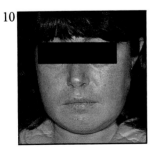

Both glucocorticoid and mineralocorticoid adrenal secretions produce hypertension. Glucocorticoids produce the characteristic appearances of Cushing's syndrome [10] which may be due to either adrenal tumours or hyperplasia. The latter may be secondary to stimulation of the adrenal glands as a result of a basophil pituitary tumour. Primary aldosteronism (Conn's syndrome [11]) results from hypersecretion of aldosterone which, in addition to producing hypertension, gives rise to a characteristic hypokalaemic alkalosis. The majority of cases of primary aldosteronism are due to a tumour but a substantial minority are caused by bilateral multinodular hyperplasia. The biochemical changes are

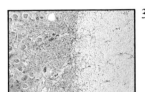

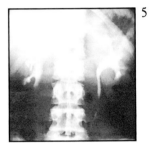

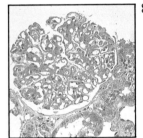

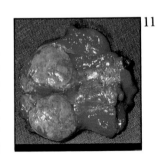

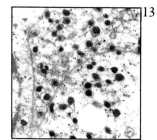

usually less marked in this condition. Adrenal medullary tumours produce hypertension through secretion of excessive amounts of the catecholamines, noradrenaline and adrenaline (phaeochromocytoma) [12]. Occasionally, these tumours may lie outside the adrenal glands, developing in sympathetic tissue in, for instance, the urinary bladder, thorax, organ of Zuckerkandl or other situations within the abdomen. These tumours are loaded with stored catecholamines [13] and manipulation, i.e. during palpation of the abdomen or during surgery, may cause the release of catecholamines and disastrous paroxysmal hypertension.

Hypertension is frequently seen in rare endocrine conditions such as acromegaly, myxoedema or hyperparathyroidism. It frequently regresses when these conditions are treated medically or surgically.

Medication

Hypertension may be iatrogenic e.g. due to steroid treatment or as a result of the contraceptive pill. A slight elevation of blood pressure is produced by medication which causes fluid retention e.g. carbenoxolone or non-steroidal antiinflammatory drugs. It can also be produced by drugs which mimic the action of the sympathetic nervous system such as ephedrine, amphetamine and monoamine oxidase inhibitors taken with tyramine containing foods. Withdrawal of clonidine may cause hypertension through increased sympathetic activity.

Hypertension of Pregnancy

Hypertension may occur in pregnancy as a result of pre-existing renal disease or essential hypertension. In addition, hypertension may occur (particularly in first pregnancies) after the thirtieth week of gestation in association with proteinuria and oedema (pre-eclamptic toxaemia). Renal biopsy in such patients has shown enlarged oedematous glomeruli with narrowing of the capillary lumina and swelling of endothelial cells [14].

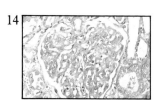

Coarctation

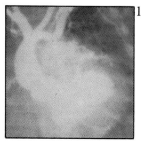

This is a congenital narrowing of the aorta usually just below the origin of the left subclavian artery, causing hypertension proximal to the lesion [15,16].

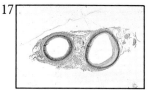

Large Arteries and Arterioles

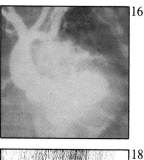

Increased perfusion pressure causes hypertrophy of the smooth muscle of the vascular media. The internal elastic lamina becomes duplicated and there is fibrous thickening of the sub-intimal part of the artery [17,18]. The aorta and larger vessels arising from it are slightly dilated and lose some of their elasticity. The peripheral large arteries may become elongated and tortuous [19] so that visible pulsations may be noticeable, particularly in older subjects. Atheroma is more frequently seen in hypertensive patients [20].

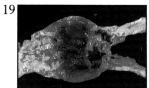

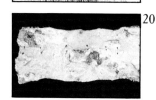

Small Arteries and Arterioles

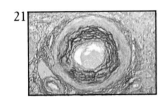

Medial hypertrophy occurs with an increased collagen content in the media [21]. Sub-intimal thickening is more pronounced and as a result the lumen of the vessel is narrowed. The increase in wall to lumen ratio in the smaller arteries and arterioles causes an increased resistance to flow and may therefore help to perpetuate and, indeed, amplify blood pressure elevation. Arterioles characteristically display hyaline thickening which develops gradually from patchy deposition until, in longstanding hypertension, it may replace the structure of the arteriolar wall leaving only the endothelium intact [22]. It is most frequently seen in the arterioles of the abdominal viscera and in the renal vessels. It is probably not of great functional significance.

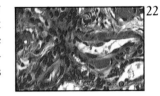

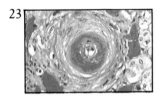

Patients with accelerated (malignant) hypertension usually have fibrinoid necrosis [23] of the smaller arteries; this arises because hypertensive damage results in increased permeability of the vascular endothelium to plasma proteins. The vessel wall is replaced by a structureless fibrin-like material containing plasma protein components. A distinct lesion, but often associated with fibrinoid necrosis, is progressive extreme intimal thickening by concentric collagenous rings (onion skinning).

The Heart

The need to contract against increased resistance produces left ventricular hypertrophy in hypertensive patients [24]. With the development of sensitive non-invasive methods such as echocardiography it has become apparent that a mild degree of left ventricular hypertrophy occurs quite early in the development of hypertension. This is not reflected in changes in the external cardiac profile but is associated with a slight reduction in cavity volume and in compliance of the left ventricle. This has important functional consequences since prognosis of hypertension is worse in patients with more marked degrees of left ventricular hypertrophy. Left ventricular failure [25] in hypertension is associated with dilatation of the left ventricle.

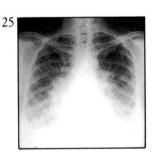

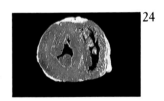

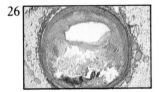

In addition to these direct consequences of increased afterload, coronary atheroma is much more frequent in hypertensive patients [26]. Myocardial infarction is the most frequent cause of death in hypertensive patients and is three times as common as stroke.

The Brain

Hypertension has both direct and indirect effects upon the brain. Increased prevalence of atheroma in both extracranial and intracranial vessels increases the risk of cerebral infarction either as a result of *in situ* thrombosis or embolization from a distant site.

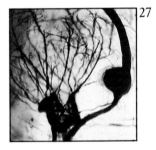

Intracerebral haemorrhage occurs as a result of rupture of a Charcot-Bouchard aneurysm [27]. These are small degenerative lesions occurring in the basal ganglia, thalamus and internal capsule. Thrombosis of these aneurysms may also give rise to small lacunar infarctions in the brain, causing minor strokes.

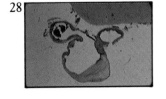

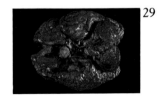

Aneurysms of the circle of Willis are congenital lesions giving rise to subarachnoid haemorrhage [28,29]. Whilst they are more

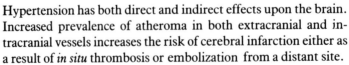

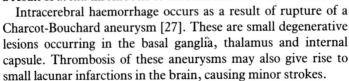

frequent in hypertensive patients, they also often cause subarachnoid haemorrhage in normotensive patients.

Sudden acute rises in cerebral perfusion pressure give rise to focal areas of vasodilatation in the smaller arteries and arterioles of the brain. The dilated areas are abnormally permeable and cause local cerebral oedema. This is the pathological basis of hypertensive encephalopathy.

The Kidneys

Renal failure is very rare in patients with essential hypertension unless they have entered the accelerated phase. Nevertheless, histological changes are evident. Atheroma of the renal vessels or renal embolization from the aorta or renal arteries may cause infarction and scarring. The renal vessels show the changes of hypertension described above. Hyaline degeneration is particularly evident, often in the afferent glomerular arterioles. The normal loss of nephrons with ageing is accelerated in essential hypertension so that histologically nephrosclerosis becomes evident. There is frequently a moderate reduction in renal size with diffuse cortical thinning [30]. Scarring of the surface of the kidney leads to an adherent capsule with an irregular sub-capsular surface. Whilst vascular disease usually produces a slight reduction in renal blood flow, glomerular filtration rate is maintained.

Both renal blood flow and glomerular filtration rate are reduced in accelerated hypertension as a result of the vascular lesions of malignant hypertension. Renal failure may progress rapidly. The afferent renal arterioles are particularly susceptible to fibrinoid necrosis. The afferent arteriole wall is disrupted, the lumen is often completely obliterated and therefore the distal glomerulus is destroyed. Since this is a relatively acute process the kidneys are usually normal in size and the sub-capsular surface is spotted with tiny haemorrhages [31].

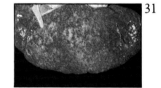

Symptoms

In the majority of patients hypertension gives rise to no symptoms until target organ damage occurs. There is, however, an increased incidence of nocturia and epistaxis in hypertensive patients. Hypertensive headaches are characteristically situated in the occiput, throbbing in character and occurring in the early morning. However, the vast majority of headaches in hypertensive patients are not attributable to high blood pressure.

Physical Signs

The pulse is usually normal in hypertensive patients. Marked left ventricular hypertrophy gives rise to a forceful displaced apex beat. The aortic component of the second sound may be accentuated and an ejection systolic murmur may be heard in the aortic area. Advanced hypertensive disease may give rise to signs of left ventricular failure or aortic regurgitation.

Fundal appearances give best assessment of the vascular tree during clinical examination. Thickening of the arterial wall gives rise to an increased reflection of light ('light reflex') and the appearance of silver wiring. The veins may be nipped at the point

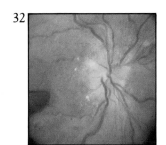

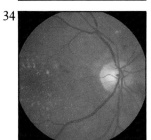

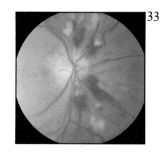

where they cross an artery (arteriovenous nipping) [32]. It should be emphasized that both these appearances occur in normotensive elderly patients and the presence of either sign is therefore of little significance in patients from their late fifties onwards. These appearances are frequently referred to as grade 1 and grade 2 retinopathy respectively. Grade 3 retinopathy is associated with haemorrhages and exudates [33]. The latter comprises two types. Hard exudates are small, discrete, white lesions caused by small amounts of denatured protein [34]. Cottonwool spots are larger white lesions with a less distinct outline. They are due to retinal infarction secondary to arterial blockage. Grade 4 changes are characterized by papilloedema. Both grade 3 and grade 4 changes are associated with a bad prognosis in the untreated patient. Recent studies have suggested that there is no difference in prognosis between grade 3 and grade 4 changes.

Investigations

Routine Tests

The vast majority of patients with essential hypertension have normal serum biochemistry. Renal impairment is usually evidence for either a renal cause of hypertension or hypertension which has entered the accelerated phase. Urine testing may also be normal. Abnormal proteinuria suggests either primary renal disease or accelerated hypertension. The latter is also associated with casts and red cells [35]. Increased numbers of white cells suggest renal parenchymal disease e.g. pyelonephritis.

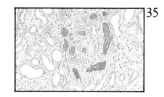

Electrocardiogram

The ECG may be normal or show left axis deviation in patients with mild hypertension in whom more sensitive investigations show significant left ventricular hypertrophy. More marked longstanding hypertension is associated with electrocardiographic evidence of left ventricular hypertrophy i.e. an increase in the R wave voltage in the left chest leads and in the S waves in the right chest leads so that the sum of the two exceeds 35 mm. Later T wave flattening, ST depression and T wave inversion occur in the antero-lateral chest leads (left ventricular strain) [36].

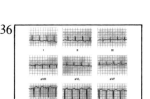

Chest X-ray

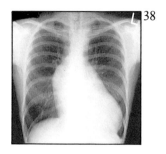

Mild to moderate hypertension is frequently associated with a normal chest X-ray. Left ventricular enlargement may be manifested by an increased cardiothoracic ratio although this is a comparatively insensitive measure. In addition, the aortic shadow becomes 'unfolded'. Left ventricular failure is manifested by a 'bats wing' appearance of the pulmonary vessels, cardiomegaly, small pleural effusions and Kerley's B-lines [37]. Rib notching may be visible in patients with coarctation of the aorta [38]. This is produced by collateral vessels by-passing the coarctation.

Renal Radiology

Intravenous urography is usually normal in patients with essen-

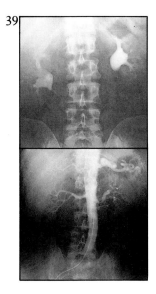

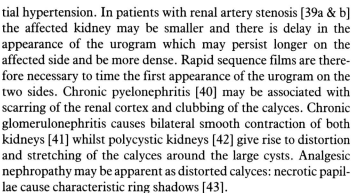

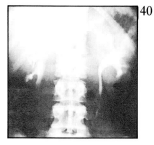

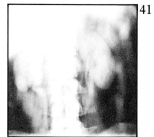

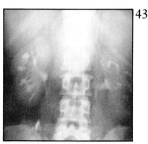

tial hypertension. In patients with renal artery stenosis [39a & b] the affected kidney may be smaller and there is delay in the appearance of the urogram which may persist longer on the affected side and be more dense. Rapid sequence films are therefore necessary to time the first appearance of the urogram on the two sides. Chronic pyelonephritis [40] may be associated with scarring of the renal cortex and clubbing of the calyces. Chronic glomerulonephritis causes bilateral smooth contraction of both kidneys [41] whilst polycystic kidneys [42] give rise to distortion and stretching of the calyces around the large cysts. Analgesic nephropathy may be apparent as distorted calyces: necrotic papillae cause characteristic ring shadows [43].

Renal angiography may be necessary to demonstrate the lesion in renal artery stenosis. Atheromatous plaques may be visible as small, discrete lesions causing luminal narrowing and post-stenotic dilatation. Fibromuscular dysplasia causes a characteristic corkscrew appearance with alternate areas of narrowing and dilatation [44]. Phaeochromocytoma can be demonstrated by arteriography. However, CAT scanning is a safer and preferable option.

Adrenal adenomata can be demonstrated by either arteriography or adrenal phlebography [45]. These lesions can also be seen on CAT scanning although they are more difficult to demonstrate.

Echocardiography

This is now the preferred non-invasive method for demonstrating left ventricular hypertrophy. It allows for measurement of both cardiac dimensions and mass and helps in the diagnosis of associated lesions such as valvular heart disease.

Ultrasonic Scanning

This may help to demonstrate transsonic renal cysts in polycystic renal disease [46] and may help in the assessment of renal size in patients with parenchymal disease.

Isotope Scanning

Radiolabelled cholesterol is taken up preferentially by the adrenal gland and used in the synthesis of adrenal steroids. This provides an excellent method for demonstrating tumours in e.g. Conn's syndrome and lateralizing them for surgery [47]. I^{131} metaiodobenzylguanethidine localizes both intra- and extra-adrenal phaeochromocytomata.

Isotope renography is useful in the demonstrating and lateralizing of renovascular disease. DTPA (technetium labelled diethylenetriamine pentaacetic acid) acts as a measure of glomerular filtration on the two sides, whilst DMSA (dimercaptosuccinic acid) or radiolabelled sodium iodohippurate serve as markers of renal plasma flow.

Nuclear Magnetic Resonance Techniques

Magnetic resonance images can be used to calculate atrial and

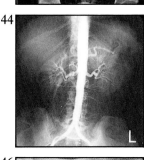

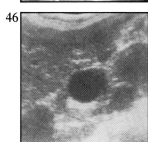

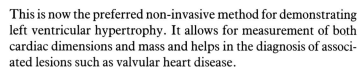

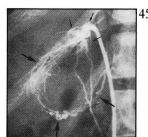

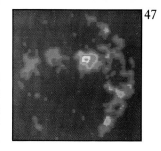

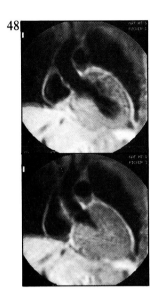

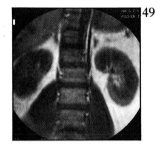

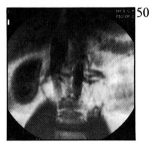

ventricular volumes and these measurements can be used to derive very accurate values for stroke volume and ejection fractions. The ventricular myocardium is well shown on magnetic resonance images and its thickness can be accurately measured [48a ,48b]. Some of the causes of hypertension, such as renal disease [49], renal artery stenosis [50] and coarctation [51] are clearly demonstrated. In addition, some of the sequelae are also seen [52]. The value of this technique in assessment of the hypertensive patient is currently a matter of research and techniques have not yet entered routine clinical practice.

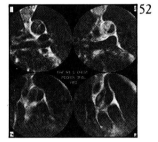

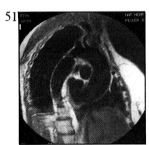

1   Systolic blood pressure distribution in healthy men and women.

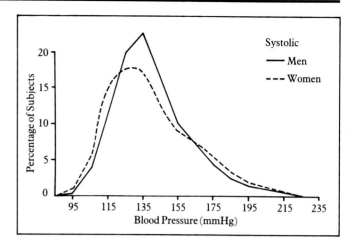

2   Left renal artery stenosis due to atheroma causing left renal atrophy and compensatory hypertrophy of the right kidney which has three patent arteries. There is mild aortic atheroma.

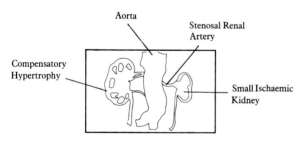

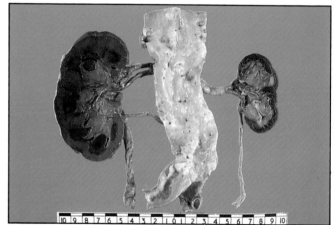

3   Long-standing renal artery stenosis has caused almost total tubular atrophy in the kidney with relative sparing of the glomeruli which are protected from the effects of systemic hypertension by the renal artery stenosis.

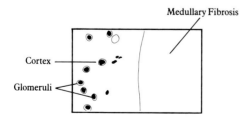

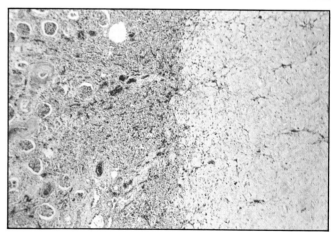

4   Large Wilm's tumour from five-year-old child
    compressing the kidney. The child presented with
    hypertension.

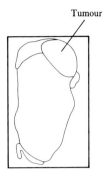

Tumour

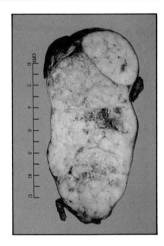

5   Intravenous urogram from hypertensive patient with
    contracted right kidney due to chronic
    pyelonephritis.

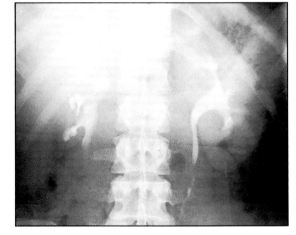

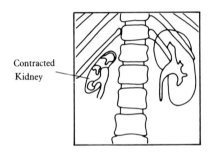

Contracted
Kidney

6   Fingers of a patient with scleroderma. The patient
    had been treated for Raynaud's disease for several
    years when she presented with a fit secondary to
    malignant hypertension. The patient died of renal
    failure two weeks later.

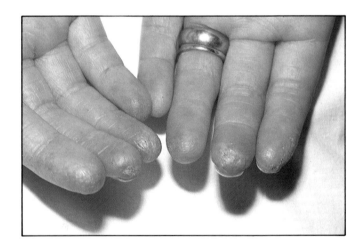

7 Proliferative glomerulonephritis. The glomerular tuft is hypercellular and swollen. Only a few glomerular capillary loops appear patent. The hypercellularity is due to increased numbers of mesangial and endothelial cells and to an infiltrate of neutrophil polymorphonuclear leucocytes. The latter are recognized by their lobed nuclei. There is no epithelial proliferation and Bowman's space remains clear.

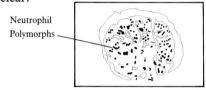

Neutrophil Polymorphs

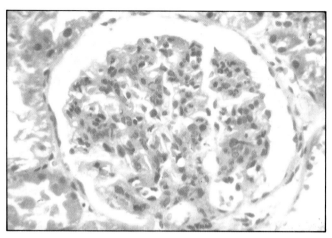

8 Advanced membranous glomerulonephritis. Resin section stained with haematoxylin and eosin shows uniform thickening of the glomerular capillaries on the edge of this biopsy. The glomerulus is of normal cellularity.

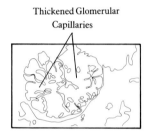

Thickened Glomerular Capillaries

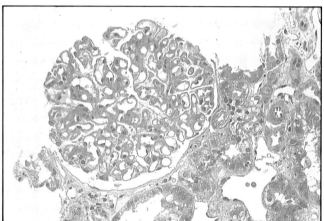

9 Minimal change glomerulonephritis. Electron micrograph from a male with nephrotic syndrome due to minimal change glomerulonephritis. There is total foot process fusion (arrows) of the epithelial cells on the outer surface of the glomerular capillary loops. There is no immune complex deposition or any other abnormality of the basement membrane.

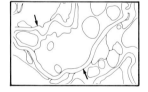

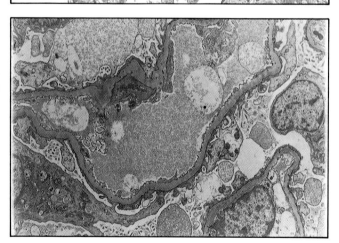

10 Facial appearance from patient who presented with moderate hypertension (BP180/110). She commented that her face had recently become rounded which had been noted by her friends. A diagnosis of Cushing's syndrome with bilateral adrenal hyperplasia was subsequently made.

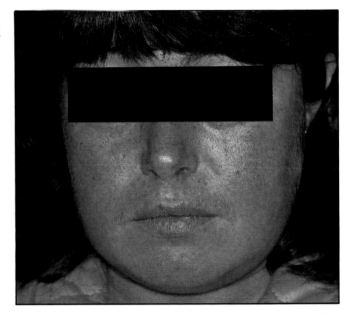

11 Adrenal gland removed at operation from a patient with primary aldosteronism. The orange tumour has been cut open.

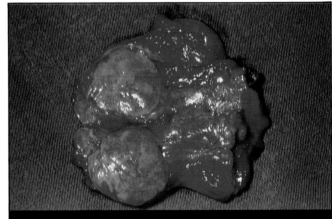

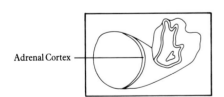

Adenoma

12 A typical adrenal phaeochromocytoma forming a round brown nodule within the medulla and quite distinct from the yellow cortical layer.

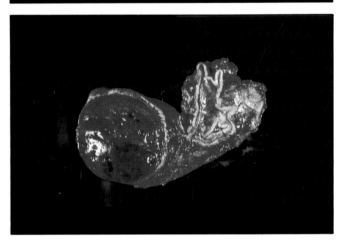

Adrenal Cortex

13 Electron micrograph ($\times$ 33,000) of phaeochromocytoma showing stored secretory granules.

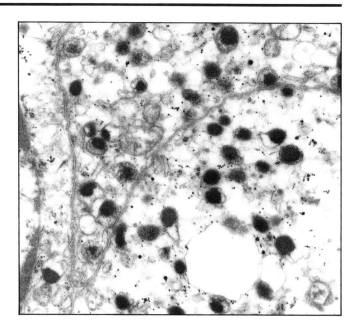

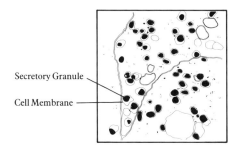

Secretory Granule

Cell Membrane

14 A swollen glomerulus from a patient dying from eclampsia shows thickening of the capillary walls due to cell swelling. The capillary loops are patent.

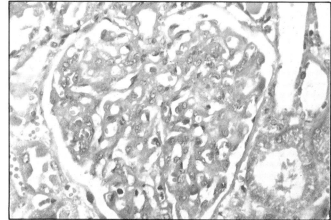

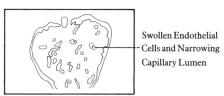

Swollen Endothelial Cells and Narrowing Capillary Lumen

15 Coarctation of the aorta just distal to the left subclavian artery. A red probe is present through the coarctation and also through a coincidental ventricular septal defect.

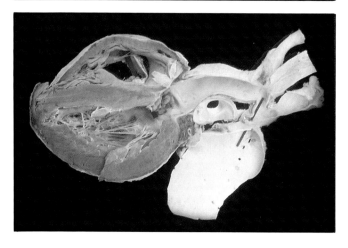

Aortic Arch

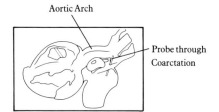

Probe through Coarctation

16 Left ventricular angiogram (antero-posterior projection) showing severe tubular hypoplasia of the aortic arch.

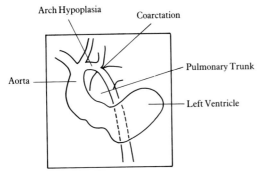

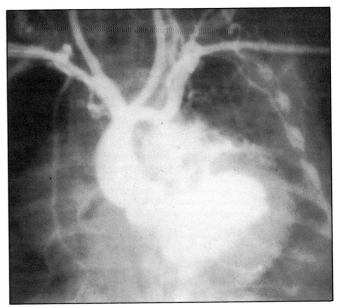

17 Carotid bifurcation showing marked intimal thickening in the sinus associated with hypertension.

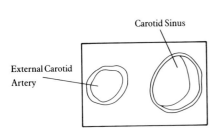

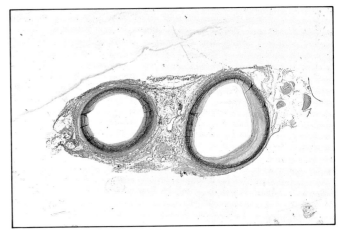

18 Higher magnification of carotid sinus wall from same patient confirming intimal thickening, irregular elastic laminae and some medial collagen increase.

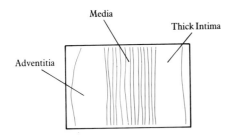

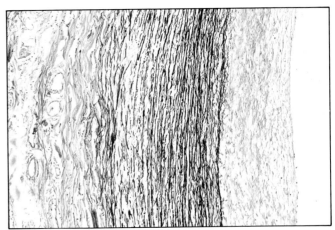

19 An atheromatous abdominal aortic aneurysm at the typical site below the renal arteries and proximal to the bifurcation. The aneurysm contains thrombus.

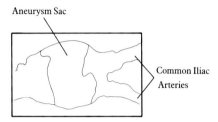

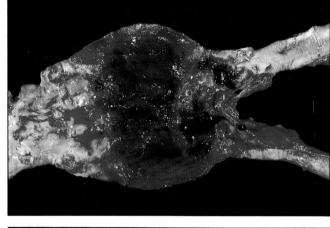

20 Aorta with severe atheroma. The plaques are ulcerated and calcified.

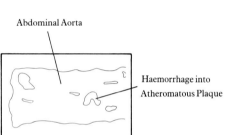

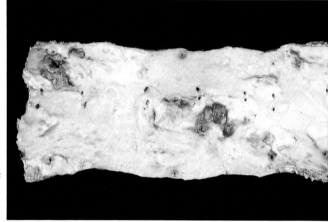

21 Section through a renal interlobular artery in essential hypertension showing reduplication of the internal elastic lamina. The lumen is reduced but patent.

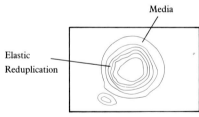

22 Microscopic appearance of hyaline arteriolar change in afferent glomerular arteriole due to essential hypertension. The hyaline deposit is sharply defined and the vessel lumen is patent.

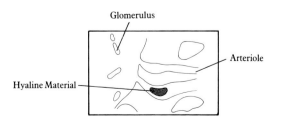

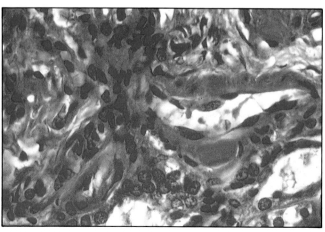

23 High power photomicrograph of renal arteriole showing fibrinoid necrosis in malignant hypertension. The fibrin deposits are blurred and poorly localized compared with the hyaline deposits in essential hypertension.

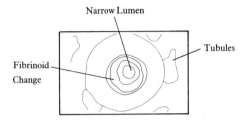

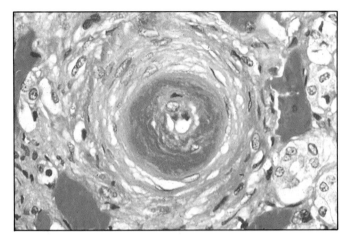

24 Transverse section of heart with concentric left ventricular hypertrophy due to hypertension. Small left ventricular cavity indicates absence of cardiac failure.

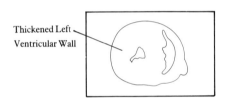

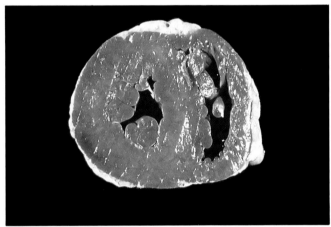

25 Chest radiograph showing pulmonary oedema and bilateral pleural effusions following acute myocardial infarction.

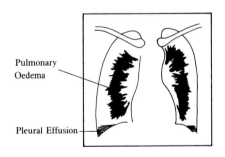

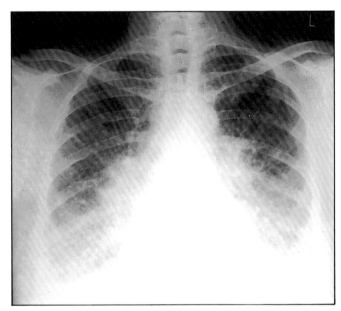

26 Transverse section of atheromatous coronary artery. The intima shows fibrous thickening with a large lipid deposit on one side leaving a reduced slit-like lumen.

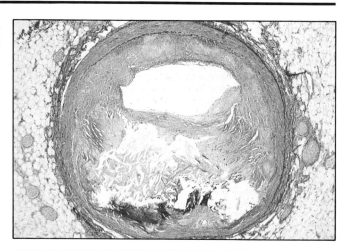

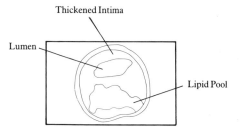

27 Charcot Bouchard aneurysm laying along the course of a small intracerebral artery

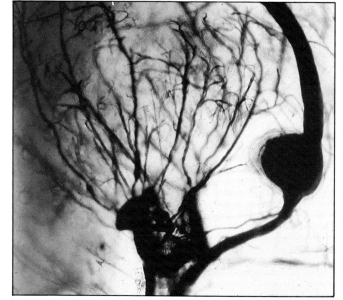

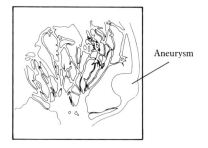

28 Microscopic section through an intact berry aneurysm on the circle of Willis. The aneurysm has a fibrous wall with no elastic tissue present.

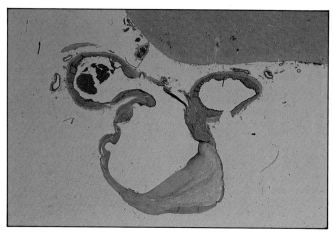

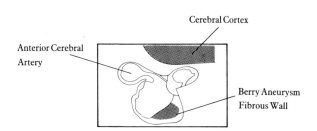

29 Inferior surface of the brain from a patient dying after extensive subarachnoid haemorrhage due to rupture of a large berry aneurysm.

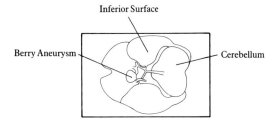

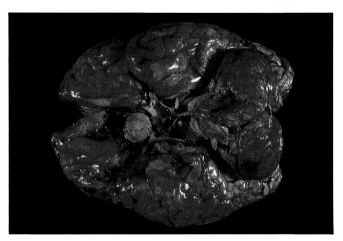

30 Nephrosclerosis due to essential hypertension causing cortical thinning with a granular capsular surface. The kidneys are atrophic due to ischaemia.

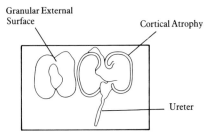

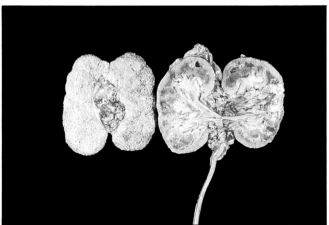

31 External surface of a kidney in malignant hypertension (BP 210/130) showing 'flea-bitten' appearance due to tiny subcapsular haemorrhages.

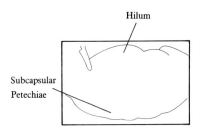

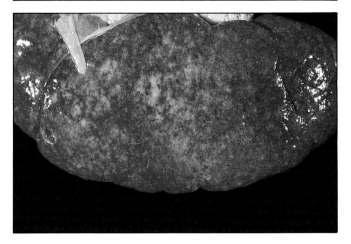

HYPERTENSION

Symptoms

32 Fundus from a hypertensive patient presenting with a subarachnoid haemorrhage. A large sub-hyaloid haemorrhage with an upper fluid level is seen on the left. There is also silver wiring with arteriovenous nipping and hard and soft exudates.

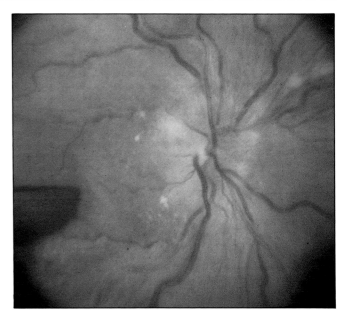

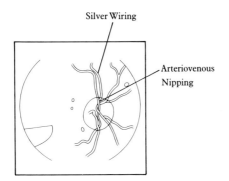

33 Fundus from a patient with malignant hypertension. Note presence of extensive haemorrhages, soft exudates and papilloedema. Blood pressure was treated medically and the patient remains well.

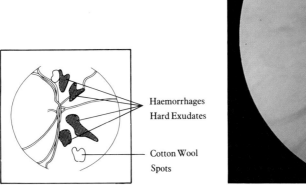

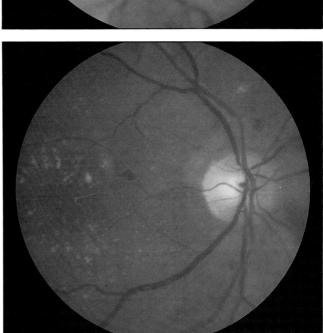

34 Fundus from a patient with accelerated hypertension. Note 'macular starring' of hard exudates and some small haemorrhages.

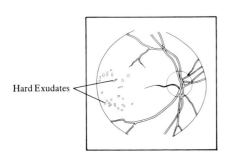

35 Red cell casts fill renal tubules and may be seen by microscopy of urine passed by patients with necrotising glomerulonephritis and some cases of malignant hypertension which cause glomerular bleeding.

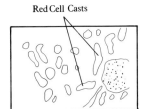

Red Cell Casts

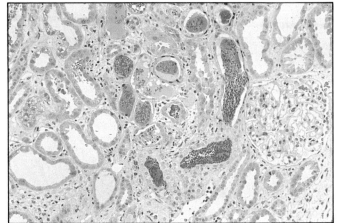

36

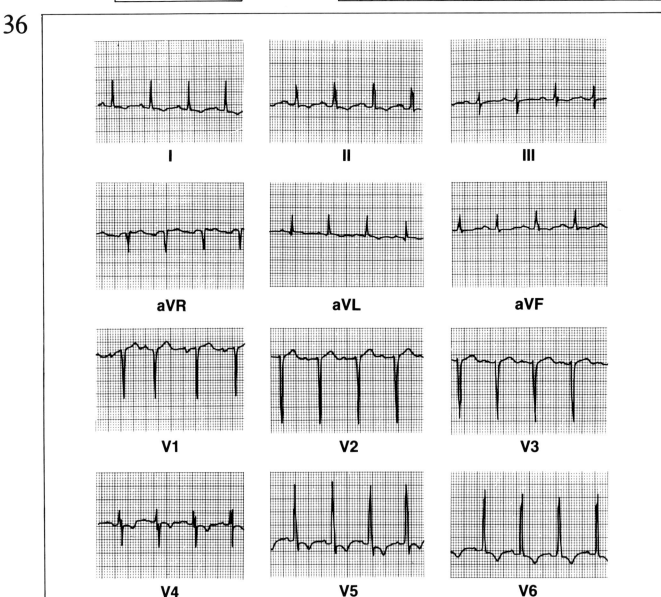

Electrocardiogram from patient with malignant hypertension. Voltage charges of left ventricular hypertrophy (deep S waves in the right ventricular leads and tall R waves in left ventricular leads) are seen together with a 'strain' pattern (inverted T waves in the left ventricular leads).

37 Chest X-ray from patient with left ventricular failure due to hypertension. Vascular engorgement gives rise to a 'bats wings' appearance and distended lymphatics cover Kerley B-lines.

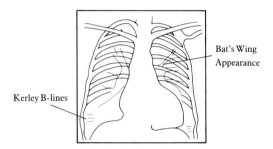

38 Chest X-ray from 20-year-old hypertensive patient. Coarctation is suggested by the rib-notching, bulging ascending aorta and absence of aorta knuckle.

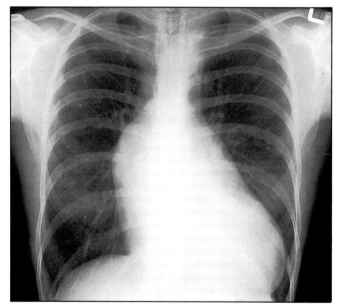

39a Intravenous urogram from patient with left renal artery stenosis at 20 minutes after injection. The dye is more concentrated in the pelvis of the left kidney.

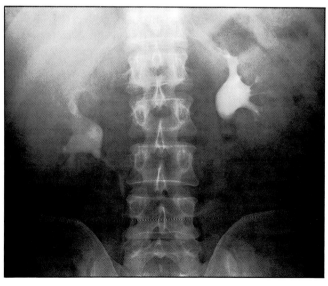

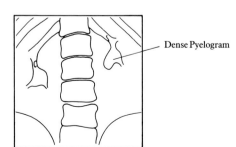

39b Renal angiogram from the same patient. A tight stenosis is seen at the mouth of the left renal artery.

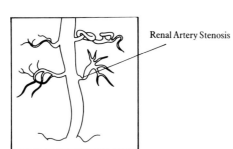

Renal Artery Stenosis

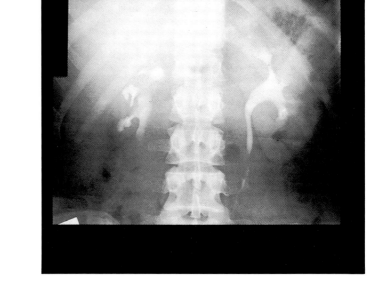

40 Intravenous urogram from hypertensive patient. Clubbing of the calyces is clearly visible on the contracted kidney.

Clubbed Calyces

41 Intravenous urogram with tomography from hypertensive patient with contracted kidneys due to chronic glomerulonephritis.

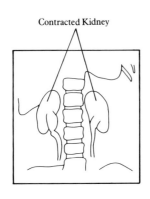

Contracted Kidney

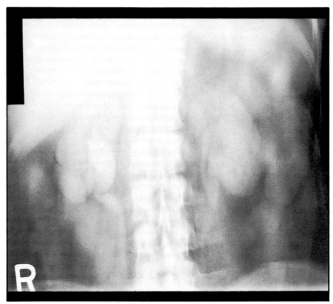

42 Intravenous urogram from patient with polycystic kidney showing calyces stretched over cysts.

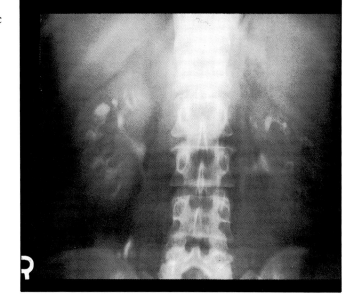

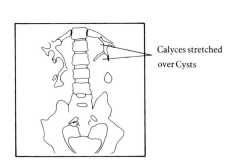

Calyces stretched over Cysts

43 Intravenous urogram from patient with papillary necrosis due to analgesic nephropathy. Characteristic 'ring' shadows are caused by necrotic papillae.

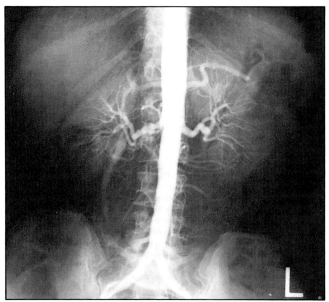

'Ring' Shadow

44 Arteriogram showing characteristic 'corkscrew' appearance from patient with fibromuscular dysplasia.

Fibromuscular Dysplasia

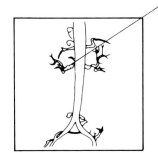

45 Right adrenal venogram from a patient with a phaeochromocytoma. The vessels are displaced by the tumour.

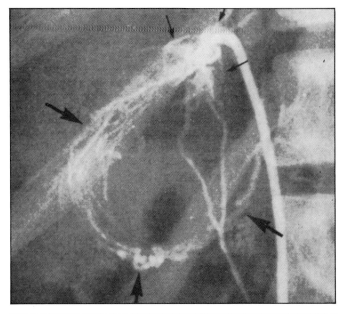

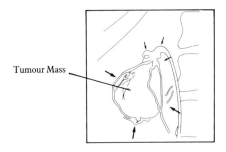

Tumour Mass

46 Ultrasound scan of kidney from patient with polycystic renal disease. Note the multiple large cysts.

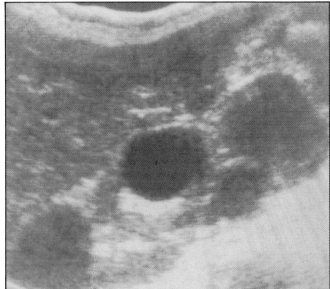

Cystic Lesions

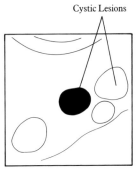

47 Isotope scan from patient with a right adrenal adenoma. Note the high concentration of isotope (shown by a brown 'hot spot' over the right adrenal).

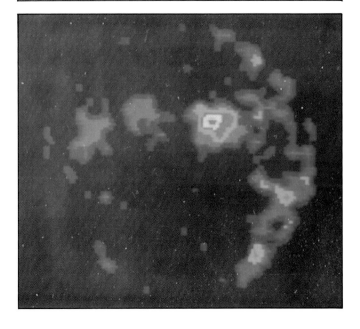

'Hot Spot'

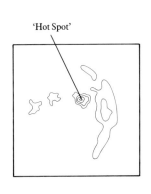

48a Left ventricular hypertrophy. Coronal image through aortic valve and left ventricle in a patient with hypertension (diastole).

DIASTOLE

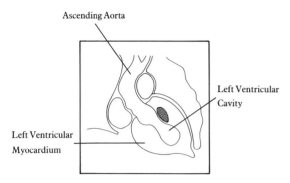

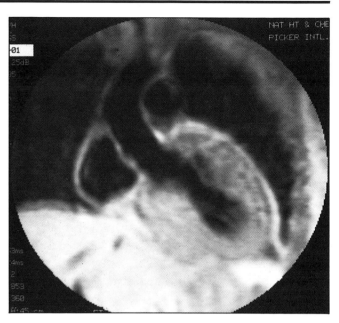

48b There is severe symmetrical hypertrophy with almost total obliteration of the left ventricular cavity at end systole (systole).

SYSTOLE

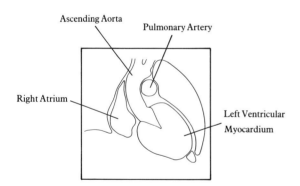

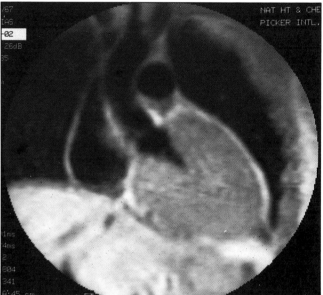

49 Normal kidneys. Coronal section through both kidneys. On the left the distinction between cortex and medulla can be seen.

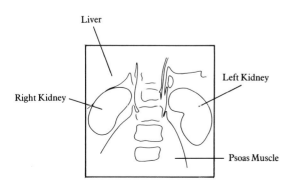

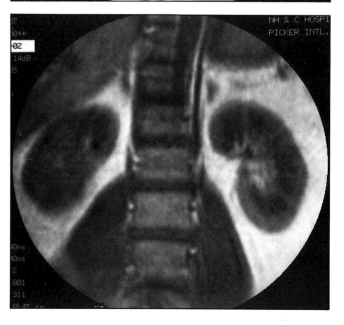

50 Renal arteries. Coronal section through the abdominal aorta showing the origins of both renal arteries. The inferior vena cava, the lower pole of the right kidney and the right ureter are also seen.

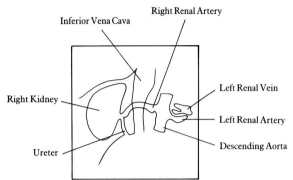

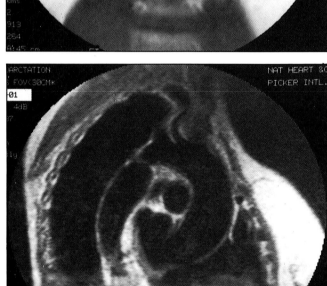

51 Coarctation. Oblique section through the aortic arch showing a coarctation just beyond the origin of the left subclavian artery.

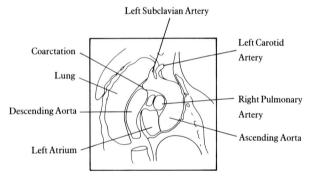

52 Dissection. Four coronal sections through the aortic arch from posterior (top left) to anterior (bottom right). There is an intimal flap dividing the lumen into true and false channels.

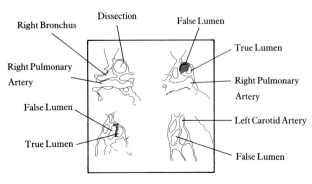

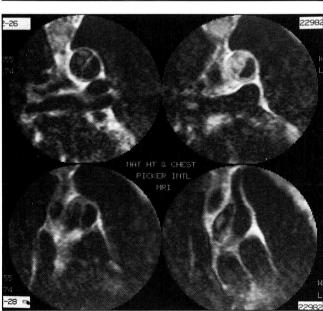

Chapter 4.
Valve Disease

Abbreviations

A	Left Atrium	FA	Femoral Artery	PE	Pericardial Effusion
a	Anterior Leaflet	IVS	Interventricular Septum	PVL	Pulmonary Valve Leaflets
Ao	Aorta	LA	Left Atrium	PVW	Posterior Ventricular Wall
Asc Ao	Ascending Aorta	LV	Left Ventricle	RA	Right Atrium
AV	Aortic Valve	LVOT	Left Ventricular Outflow Tract	RV	Right Ventricle
AVL	Aortic Valve Leaflets	MV	Mitral Valve	TV	Tricuspid Valve
CW	Chest Wall	MVL	Mitral Valve Leaflets	TVL	Tricuspid Valve Leaflets
Desc Ao	Descending Aorta	p	Posterior Leaflet	V	Left Ventricle
Eff	Effusion	P-A	Postero-Anterior	Veg	Vegetation
F	Flap	PAWP	Pulmonary Artery Wedge Pressure		

RHEUMATIC MITRAL VALVE DISEASE

Pathology

Rheumatic fever in the acute phase is characterized by inflammation in all layers of the heart: pericarditis, myocarditis and endocarditis. The pericarditis is non-specific with an acute fibrinous exudate. Myocarditis has a specific histological picture typified by the presence of Aschoff bodies, which are microscopic foci of degenerate collagen surrounded by giant cells. The pertinent features of endocarditis are small flat vegetations [1] on the closure lines of the mitral and aortic valve cusps. Microscopically the valve cusps are inflamed and thickened, the vegetations consisting largely of platelets.

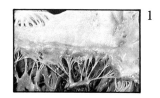

Patients who recover from the acute phase of rheumatic fever can develop chronic effects. These are seen most prominently in the endocardium. In some instances repeated sub-clinical attacks of rheumatic fever lead to progressive damage. In other patients, changes secondary to ageing and abnormal haemodynamics lead to progressive destruction of the damaged valve.

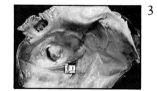

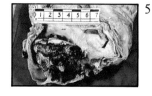

In chronic rheumatic mitral valve disease, fusion of the anterior and posterior commissures leads to a steady reduction in the area of the aperture of the fully open valve [2,3]. In some instances the valve cusps, although fused at the commissures, remain mobile. Other patients develop considerable cusp fibrosis or calcification with resultant rigidity [4]. Chronic rheumatic valve disease also produces chordal shortening and thickening. In some instances the chordae fuse into a solid fibrous mass attaching the cusps directly onto the papillary muscles. Chordal shortening decreases cusp mobility with resultant mitral regurgitation which is present in many cases of dominant stenosis. Pure regurgitation is unusual.

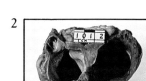

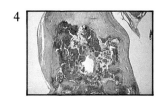

Increased left atrial pressure usually produces chamber enlargement, although there is considerable individual variation. Thrombosis may form in large atria particularly in the appendage [5]. This may be the source of systemic emboli.

Presentation

Symptoms

The main symptom is breathlessness on exertion which is caused by the rise in left atrial pressure with a consequent rise in pulmonary venous pressure. Breathlessness develops gradually in about 50% of patients. Some patients may remain asymptomatic for many years and then develop symptoms usually with the onset of atrial fibrillation. When the mitral stenosis is severe the patient may develop orthopnoea and paroxysmal nocturnal dyspnoea.

Haemoptysis occurs in about 15% of patients with mitral stenosis. There are several possible causes. The patient may bleed into the alveoli during an acute attack of pulmonary oedema; the sputum may be bloodstained during the course of intercurrent bronchitis or pneumonia; a major pulmonary vein may rupture into a bronchus owing to a considerable rise in pulmonary venous pressure; finally, haemoptysis may be produced by pulmonary infarction as a result of pulmonary embolism.

Many patients with mitral stenosis first present when embolisation from the left atrium into the systemic circulation leads to cerebral infarction, impairment of circulation to a limb, mesenteric infarction or infarction of the spleen, kidney or retina.

Palpitation may be a presenting feature in patients with rheumatic heart disease, usually when the rhythm of the heart has changed to atrial fibrillation.

Fatigue resulting from a low fixed cardiac output is a very common complaint of the patient with severe mitral stenosis.

Signs

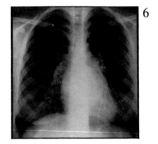

The patient may have cyanotic patches over the cheeks - the so-called mitral facies. The arterial pulse is usually normal in quality and the rhythm is frequently atrial fibrillation. If sinus rhythm is present the jugular venous pulse may show an abnormal 'a' wave due to pulmonary hypertension. Severe pulmonary hypertension may give rise to right ventricular hypertrophy and subsequent dilatation with resultant tricuspid regurgitation characterized by a dominant systolic wave in the jugular venous pulse.

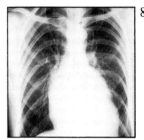

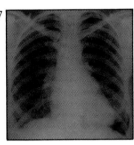

The loud first heart sound characteristic of mitral stenosis may be palpable giving rise to the 'tapping apex beat'. In addition right ventricular hypertrophy may be elicited by palpation at the left sternal edge.

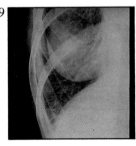

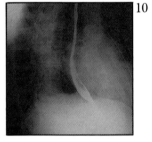

In pure mitral stenosis in sinus rhythm the auscultatory findings include an atrial systolic murmur (pre-systolic murmur) a loud first heart sound, an opening snap and variable length mid diastolic murmur. The more severe the stenosis, the closer the interval between aortic valve closure and the opening snap and the longer the mid-diastolic murmur. If the valve is calcified and rigid the first heart sound and opening snap may not be heard. If there is additional mitral regurgitation a high frequency pansystolic murmur will be heard. The presence of severe pulmonary hypertension will give rise to a loud pulmonary valve closure sound best heard at the left sternal edge but this needs to be distinguished from the opening snap which may also be best heard at the left sternal edge. If there is additional aortic or tricuspid rheumatic valve disease the physical signs of these valve lesions will be superadded or even may dominate the clinical picture.

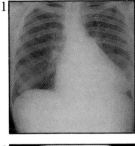

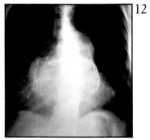

Radiology

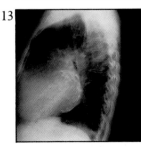

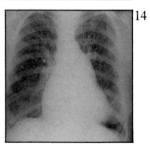

The plain chest radiograph shows left atrial enlargement [6]. Typically in mitral stenosis a prominent left atrial appendage is also seen [7]. If pulmonary venous pressure is elevated (as is usual), the upper zone vessels are dilated [8]. A higher pressure in the pulmonary veins produces septal lines and pleural effusions [7,9]. With chronic disease the valve frequently becomes calcified [10]. In long-standing cases haemosiderin deposits may be found in the lungs, seen as wide-spread mottling [11]. In patients with mixed stenosis and regurgitation the left atrium may become very large and calcified [12,13]. Long-standing pulmonary venous hypertension gives rise to pulmonary arterial hypertension. This is reflected in a large pulmonary trunk and a greater discrepancy in size between the large upper zone and the smaller lower zone vessels [14].

Electrocardiography

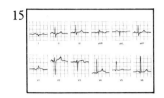

In sinus rhythm, the electrocardiogram usually shows a broad P wave in lead II, and a negative deflection in V1 reflecting left atrial enlargement [15]. Atrial fibrillation is common. Right axis deviation, tall R waves in V1 and deep S waves in V5 indicate right ventricular hypertrophy which may be present with sinus rhythm [15] or with atrial fibrillation.

Echocardiography

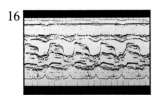

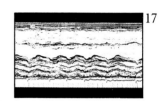

Commissural fusion produces abnormal movement of the posterior mitral valve cusp. On the M-mode echocardiogram it is seen to move forward in diastole, in the same direction as the anterior leaflet, instead of posteriorly and away from the anterior cusp [16]. The thickened leaflets return stronger echoes than normal and when calcification is present, characteristic multiple dense echoes are seen [17]. A mobile valve has a normal amplitude of excursion, but when fibrosed or calcified this is reduced. Heavy calcification and reduced mobility are reliable signs of severe disease. The two-dimensional echocardiogram enables direct visualization of the abnormal valve and its deranged movement [18].

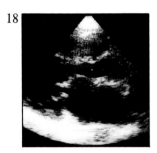

The altered pattern of inflow of blood into the left ventricle is associated with a reduction in the diastolic closure rate of the anterior mitral valve leaflet seen on the M-mode. In clinically significant mitral stenosis the diastolic closure rate is almost invariably less than 30 mm/sec.

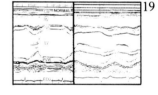

The left ventricular dimensions and septal motion are normal in mitral stenosis unless there is additional tricuspid incompetence, when septal motion may be neutral or reversed in association with an increased right ventricular dimension. In severe mitral stenosis left ventricular dimension increases in diastole more slowly than normal [19]. When there is significant mitral regurgitation the left ventricle is enlarged but fractional shortening in systole remains normal unless there is additional left ventricular disease.

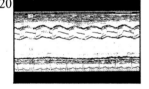

Enlargement of the left atrium is also seen on the echocardiogram [20].

Cardiac Catheterization and Angiography

Unless information about the coronary arteries is required, cardiac catheterization is unnecessary in most cases of rheumatic mitral valve disease. An individual patient can be assessed on the basis of the clinical features and non-invasive investigation and the need for surgery so determined.

In a typical case of mitral stenosis left atrial pressure will be raised depending on the severity of the stenosis and the compliance of the left atrium. The elevation of the pulmonary artery pressure may reflect the rise in left atrial pressure or additional rise in pulmonary vascular resistance. The pressure difference across the mitral valve may be determined from simultaneous left atrial (or pulmonary capillary wedge pressure) and left ventricular diastolic pressures and knowledge of cardiac output will enable mitral valve orifice size to be calculated.

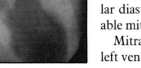

Mitral regurgitation when present can be roughly assessed by left ventricular angiography [21].

1   Mitral valve in the acute phase of rheumatic fever showing the characteristic row of small sessile vegetations along the line of closure.

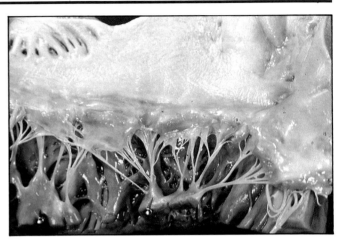

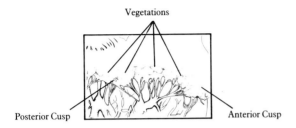

2   Fully open normal mitral and tricuspid valves viewed from left and right atria.

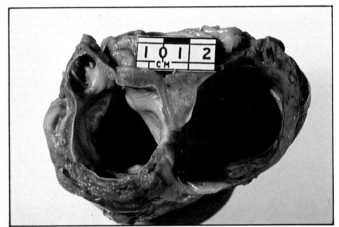

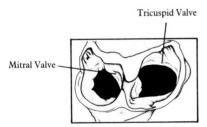

3   Rheumatic mitral stenosis viewed from left atrium. The valve orifice is a small crescentic fixed opening. The atrium is enlarged. Some calcification is present in the anterior cusp.

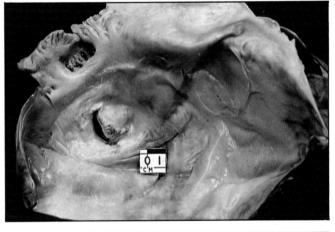

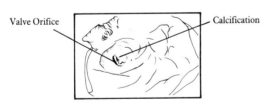

4   Histology of a rheumatic mitral valve. The valve is thickened with masses of dystrophic calcification.

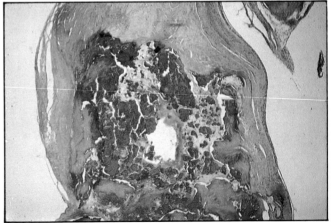

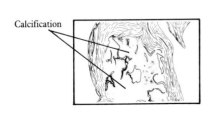

5 Typical mitral stenosis viewed from left atrium. The valve orifice is a small oval. A large mass of thrombus almost fills the atrium arising from the left atrial appendage.

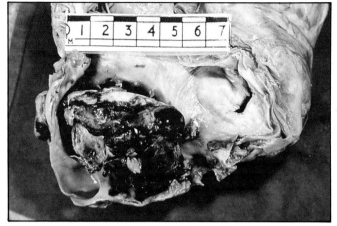

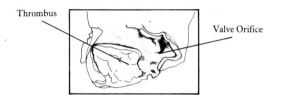

RHEUMATIC MITRAL VALVE DISEASE

Radiology

6 Chest radiograph showing left atrial enlargement.

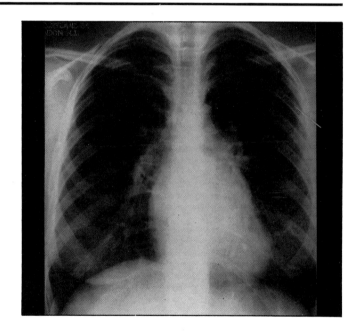

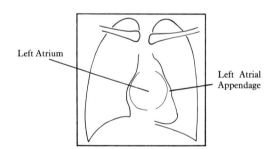

7 Chest radiograph showing small heart with a large left atrial appendage. There are bilateral pleural effusions.

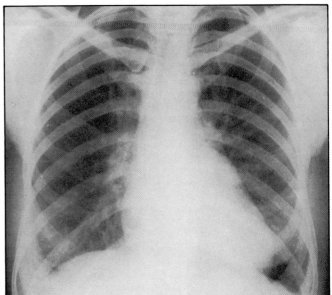

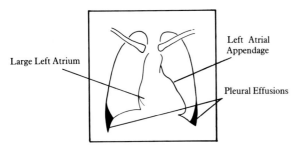

8 Chest radiograph of a patient with mitral valve disease showing [1] enlargement of left atrium, [2] distended upper lobe pulmonary veins, [3] constricted lower lobe veins.

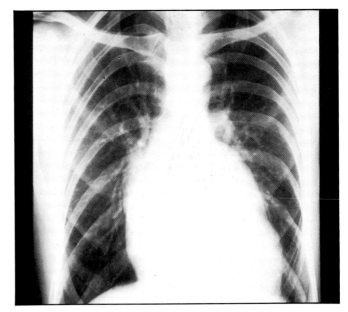

9 Detail from chest radiograph showing septal lines and pleural effusion.

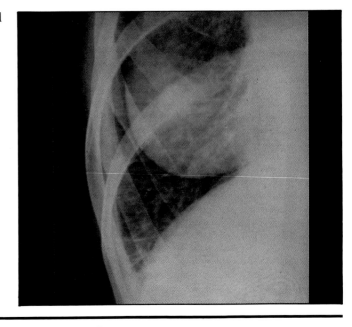

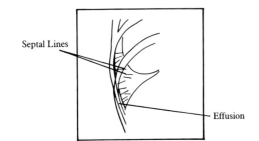

10 Chest radiograph (oblique projection) with barium outlining the oesphagus showing calcification of the mitral valve.

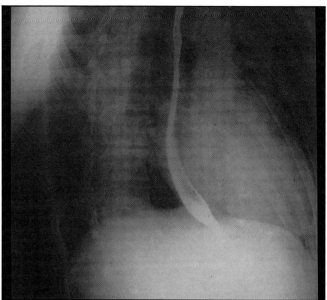

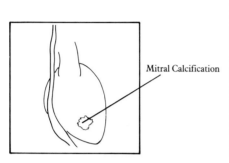

Mitral Calcification

11 Chest radiograph showing typical fine mottling of haemosiderosis.

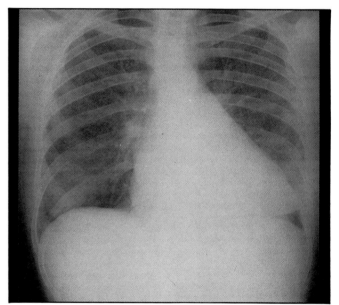

Fine Mottling

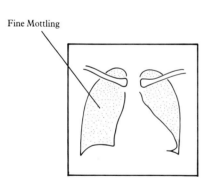

12 Chest radiograph (penetrated P-A view) showing a very large, calcified left atrium.

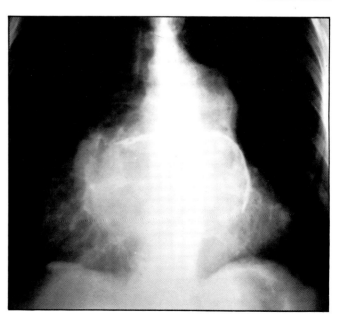

Calcified left atrium

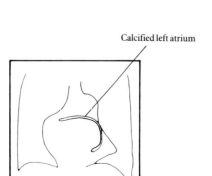

13 Chest radiograph (lateral projection) from same patient as fig.12 showing calcified left atrium.

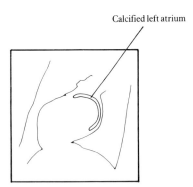

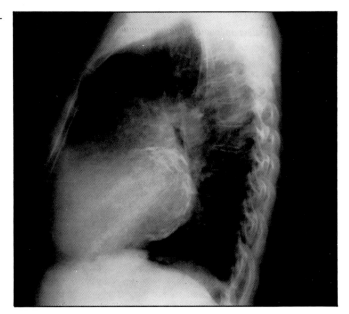

14 Chest radiograph showing a large pulmonary trunk and upper zone vessels. Lower segmental vessels are small.

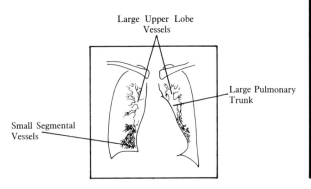

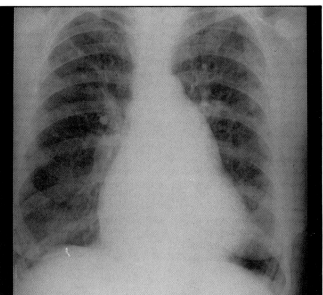

15

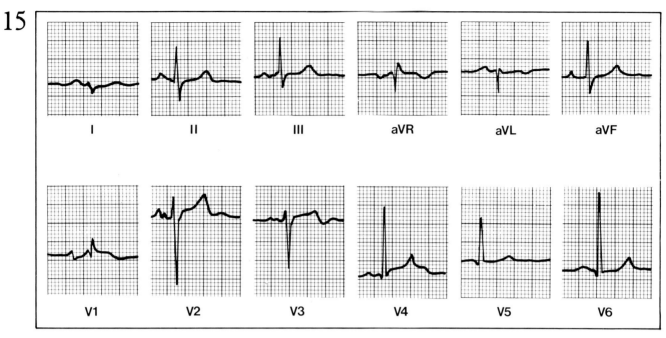

Electrocardiogram of moderately severe mitral stenosis showing the broad bifid P wave of left atrial enlargement (P mitrale), right ventricular hypertrophy as shown by a dominant R wave in lead V1. Note for V3 to V5 1mv = 0.5cm.

RHEUMATIC MITRAL VALVE DISEASE

Echocardiography

16

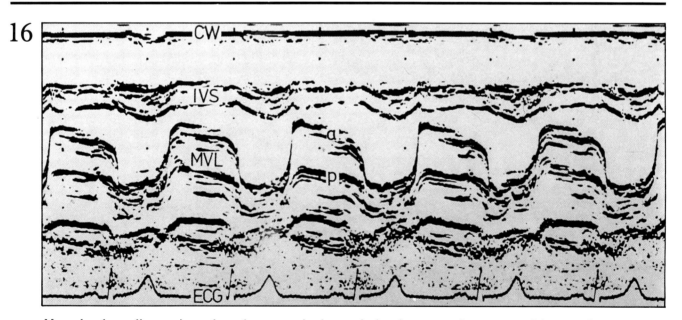

M-mode echocardiogram in moderately severe mitral stenosis showing reversed movement of the posterior cusp. The diastolic closure rate is reduced and no re-opening is seen after atrial systole.

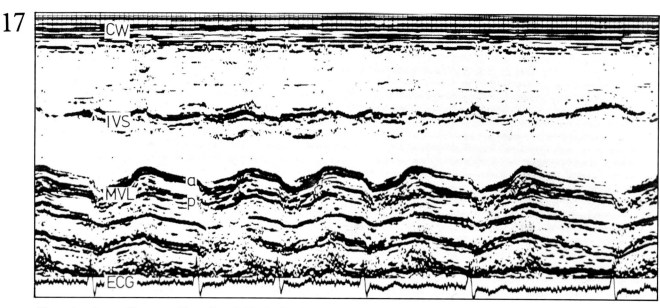

M-mode echocardiogram of heavily calcified mitral valve showing multiple echoes, reversed posterior cusp movement and reduced amplitude of movement of the anterior cusp.

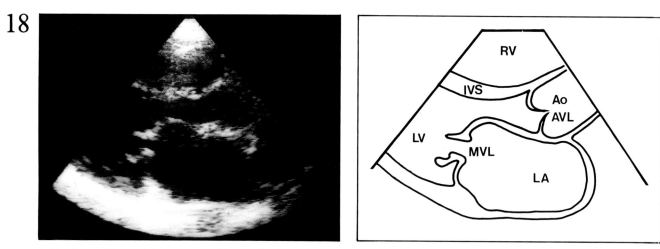

2-D echocardiographic parasternal long axis view of a stenotic mitral valve during diastole. Note the thickening of the leaflet tips and the doming of the anterior leaflet.

19

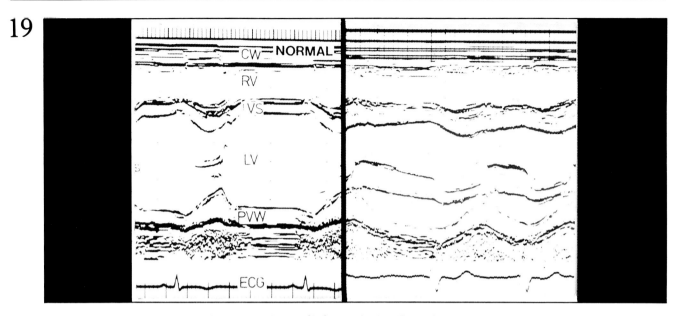

M-mode echocardiogram showing reduced rate of left ventricular dimension increase in diastole in a patient with mitral stenosis (right). Compare with normal (left).

20

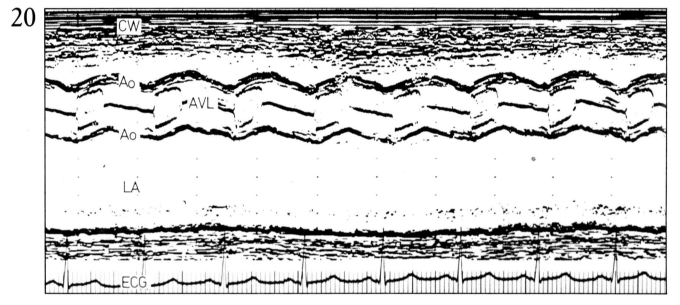

M-mode echocardiogram in mitral stenosis showing left atrial enlargement (6cm). The rate of posterior aortic root movement is reduced.

21 Left ventricular angiogram (right anterior oblique projection) showing slight mitral regurgitation through a stenotic valve.

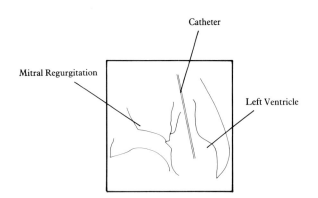

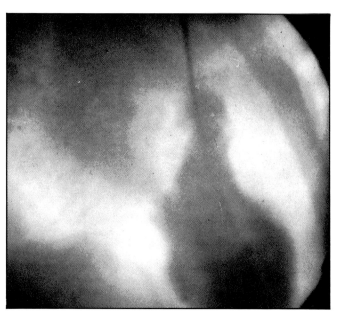

MITRAL REGURGITATION (NON-RHEUMATIC)

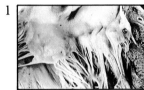

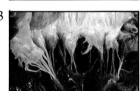

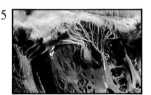

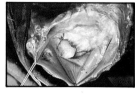

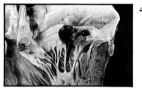

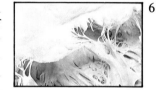

Pathology

The competence of the mitral valve depends upon the normal co-ordinated function of the left atrial wall, mitral annulus, leaflets, chordae tendineae, papillary muscles and left ventricular myocardium. Disease may affect any one or all of these structures and result in mitral regurgitation. Redundant cusp tissue and elongation of the chordae tendineae can result in a floppy mitral valve permitting slight mitral regurgitation to occur [1,2]. More severe regurgitation may develop over a long period or may occur acutely if there is chordal rupture spontaneously [3] or as a result of infective endocarditis [4].

In patients with coronary artery disease, infarction involving a papillary muscle may lead to its rupture with the development of sudden severe mitral regurgitation [5]. Ischaemia of the papillary muscles can cause long standing disorganisation of the subvalvular mitral apparatus with resultant mitral regurgitation [6]. Mitral regurgitation may be secondary to left ventricular myocardial disease, such as dilated cardiomyopathy, as a result of stretching the mitral annulus. It may also occur in left ventricular myocardial disease due to coronary atheroma when regional abnormalities of left ventricular function develop, which interfere with the subvalvular apparatus.

Presentation

Symptoms

Patients with slight mitral regurgitation, due for example to floppy mitral valve, are usually asymptomatic although rarely patients will complain of non-specific chest pain or palpitation due to various arrhythmias. When long-standing mitral regurgitation is severe and pulmonary venous pressure significantly raised, the patient will develop dyspnoea due to the marked rise in pulmonary venous pressure.

Signs

Unless mitral regurgitation is severe the carotid pulse will be normal. With long-standing significant mitral regurgitation, atrial fibrillation may develop. The reduction in cardiac output in severe cases will result in a small carotid pulse with a sharp upstroke. With the development of pulmonary hypertension and the retention of sinus rhythm the jugular venous pressure may show a dominant 'a' wave. In chronic, moderate or severe mitral regurgitation the apical impulse is hyperdynamic due to the increased stroke volume of the left ventricle unless the cause of the regurgitation is left ventricular myocardial disease.

Prolapse of a leaflet of the mitral valve into the left atrium at peak left ventricular systolic pressure gives rise to a mid or late systolic click. The subsequent slight mitral regurgitation will give rise to a late systolic murmur. Irrespective of cause, if the valve is incompetent throughout the whole of systole there will be a pansystolic murmur. Shortening of left ventricular ejection results in an abnormally wide but physiologically split second heart sound. The pulmonary component will be accentuated if there is additional pulmonary hypertension. Rapid left ventricular filling of an increased volume of blood is associated with a third heart sound.

Investigations

Radiology

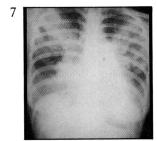

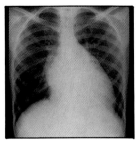

Acute severe mitral regurgitation due to chordal rupture results in pulmonary oedema which is evident on the chest radiograph often with little or no cardiac enlargement [7]. If mitral regurgitation is long-standing, the chest radiograph shows cardiac enlargement with left atrial dilatation indistinguishable from chronic rheumatic mitral valve disease [8]. Dilatation of the upper lobe pulmonary veins will reflect long-standing elevation in pulmonary venous pressure.

Electrocardiography

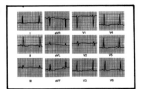

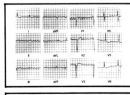

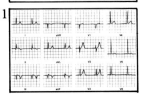

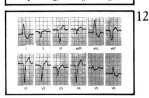

In a patient with a floppy mitral valve with only slight regurgitation or in acute severe regurgitation due to chordal rupture, the electrocardiogram may be normal or show minor ST-T abnormalities in the infero-lateral leads [9]. In chronic severe regurgitation there may be atrial fibrillation and increased left ventricular voltage with or without ST-T changes [10]. In acute rupture of the papillary muscle the ECG may show acute inferior myocardial infarction [11]. In patients with secondary mitral regurgitation from left ventricular myocardial disease, the ECG often shows left bundle branch block [12].

Echocardiography

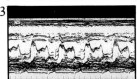

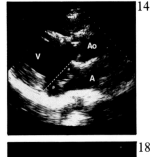

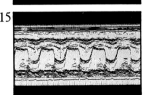

Echocardiography allows the motion of the mitral valve to be visualised and consequently distinguishes between valvular abnormalities due to rheumatic involvement and mitral regurgitation of non-rheumatic aetiology. Prolapse of the posterior or anterior leaflet of the mitral valve is often detected by echocardiography [13,14]. More severe mitral regurgitation with a flail leaflet may also be identified [15,16]. In infective endocarditis leading to mitral regurgitation, vegetations may be seen on the mitral valve leaflets [17,18].

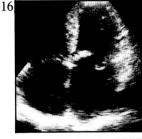

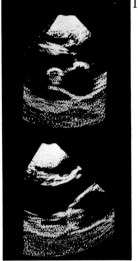

It is important to examine left ventricular systolic function in patients with mitral regurgitation; the large left ventricular stroke volume with normal ventricular contraction of the patient with long-standing severe regurgitation due to mitral valve leaflet and chordal abnormalities [19] can be distinguished from the dilated but poorly contracting ventricle of the patient who has left ventricular myocardial disease such as a dilated cardiomyopathy with secondary mitral regurgitation [20,21].

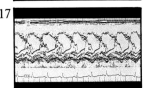

Cardiac Catheterization and Angiography

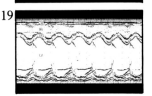

In acute severe mitral regurgitation the left atrial or pulmonary capillary wedge pressure pulse shows a large systolic 'V' wave [22]. Left ventricular angiography may demonstrate an abnormality of the mitral leaflets [23]. Chordal rupture may also be inferred if excessive movement of the leaflet is seen. In chronic severe mitral regurgitation, left ventricular dilatation may be

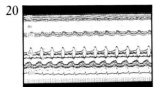

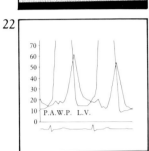

seen. Systolic function will be preserved if the cause of the regurgitation is a chordal or leaflet abnormality, but it will be impaired if the cause is left ventricular myocardial disease which may be generalised in dilated cardiomyopathy, or show regional functional abnormalities in coronary artery disease.

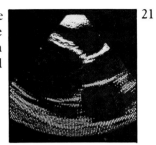

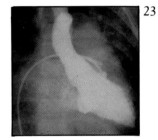

1   Mitral valve in Marfan's syndrome. Both anterior and posterior cusps are increased in area and the surface appears folded. Chordae are elongated.

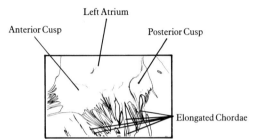

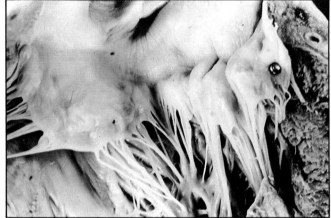

2   Floppy mitral valve viewed from the left atrium. A portion of the posterior cusp is domed into the atrium (prolapsed cusp).

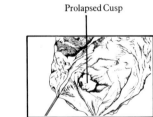

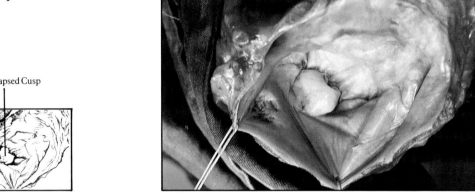

3   Floppy mitral valve with ruptured chordae. The posterior cusp is domed upward into the atrium. Stumps of ruptured chordae are present.

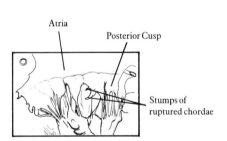

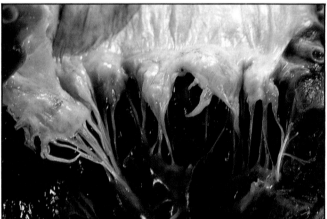

4   Mitral valve with ruptured chordae due to infective endocarditis. The posterior cusp is covered by a mass of thrombotic vegetations. Stumps of ruptured chordae are present.

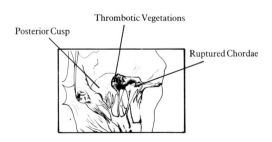

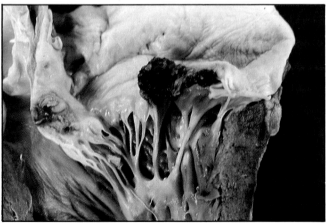

5   Partial avulsion of a papillary muscle during acute myocardial infarction producing mitral regurgitation. One head of the postero-medial papillary muscle is torn from the ventricular wall.

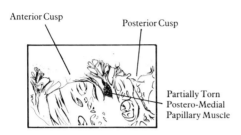

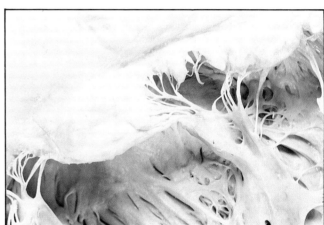

6   Fibrosis and shrinkage of the papillary muscles resulting in mitral regurgitation following myocardial infarction. The apex of the postero-medial papillary muscle is elongated and the body of the muscle is shrunken. A small chord has avulsed from the papillary muscle.

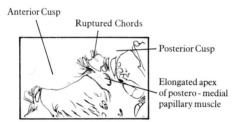

MITRAL REGURGITATION (NON-RHEUMATIC)
Radiology

7   Chest radiograph in acute chordal rupture. The heart is normal in size but there is gross pulmonary oedema.

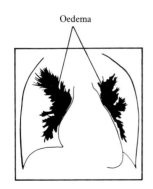

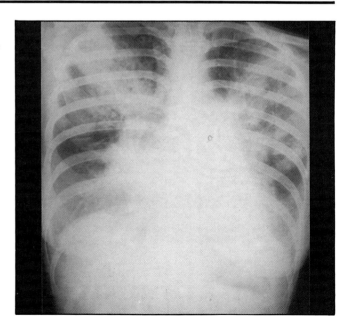

8 Chest radiograph in chronic mitral regurgitation showing cardiac enlargement, dilatation of the left atrium and the upper lobe pulmonary veins.

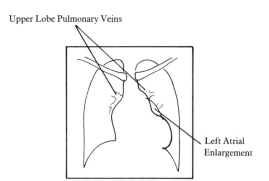

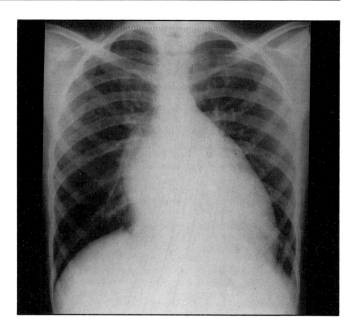

MITRAL REGURGITATION (NON-RHEUMATIC)

Electrocardiography

9

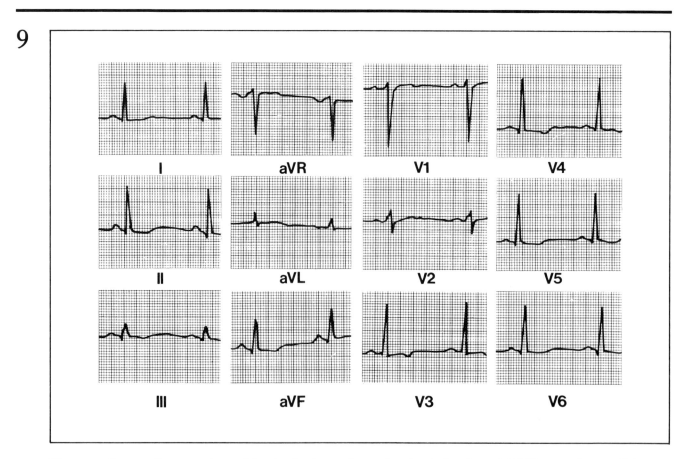

I	aVR	V1	V4
II	aVL	V2	V5
III	aVF	V3	V6

Electrocardiogram from a patient with mitral valve prolapse showing infero-lateral ST-T wave abnormalities.

10

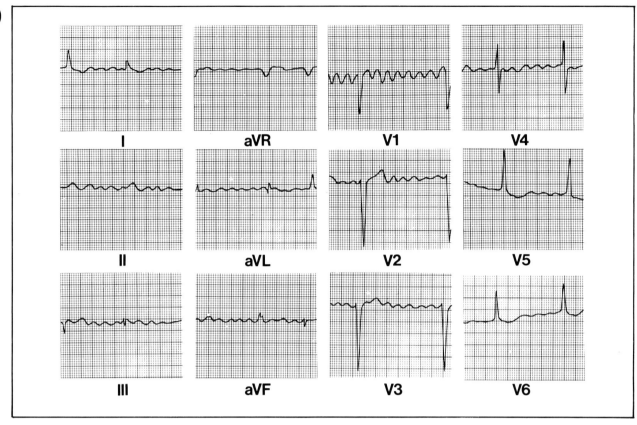

Electrocardiogram from a patient with long standing non-rheumatic mitral regurgitation showing atrial fibrillation and left ventricular hypertrophy.

11

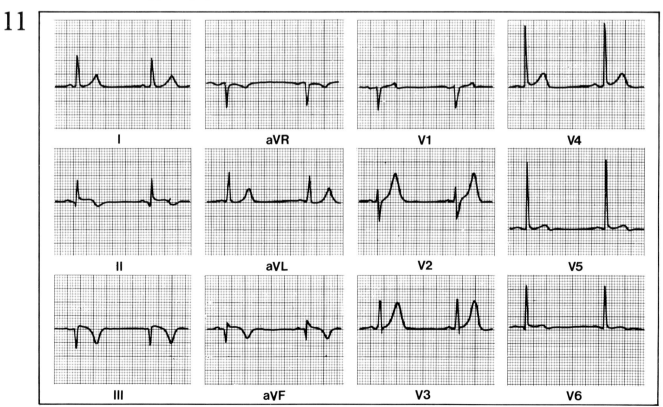

Electrocardiogram from a patient with acute papillary muscle rupture showing inferior myocardial infarction.

12

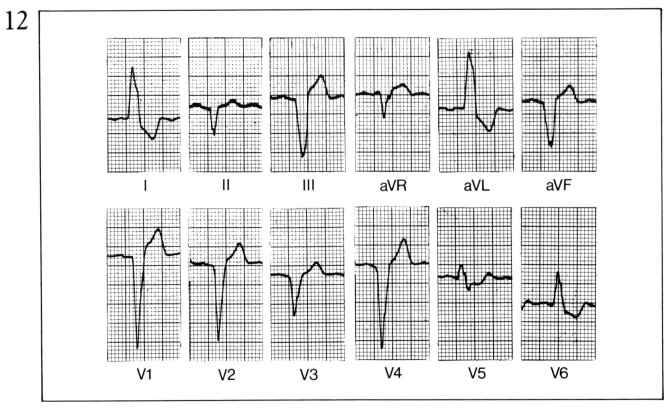

Electrocardiogram showing left bundle branch block in a patient with chronic mitral regurgitation due to dilated cardiomyopathy.

MITRAL REGURGITATION (NON-RHEUMATIC)

Echocardiography

13

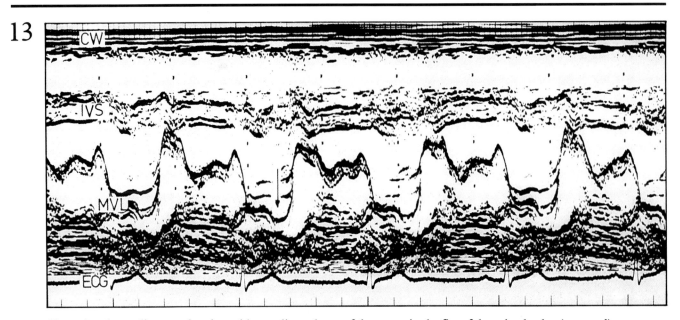

M-mode echocardiogram showing mid-systolic prolapse of the posterior leaflet of the mitral valve (arrowed).

14

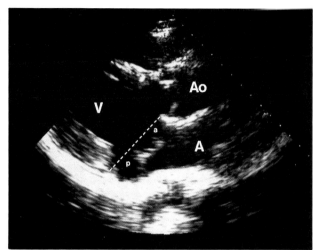 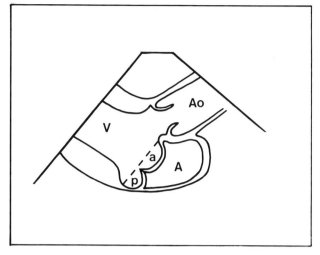

Systolic long axis 2-D echocardiographic view in mitral valve prolapse. The dotted line indicates the plane of mitral valve ring with prolapse of both anterior (a) and posterior (p) leaflets into the left atrium.

15

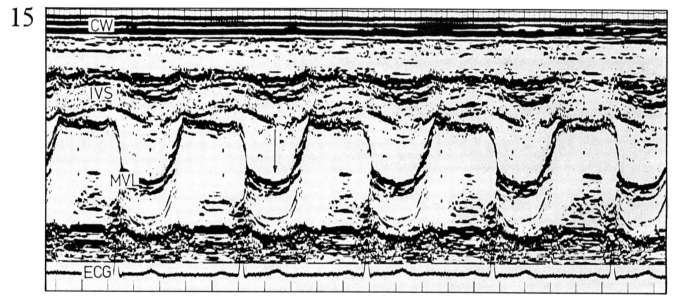

M-mode echocardiogram showing a 'hammock' prolapse of the posterior leaflet of the mitral valve (arrowed).

16

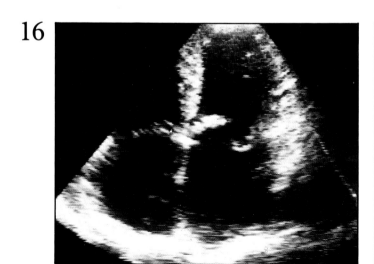 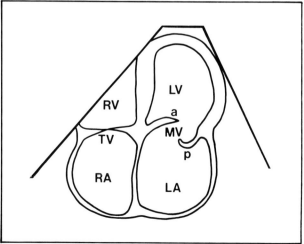

Four-chamber 2-D echocardiographic view, showing failure of coaptation of anterior and posterior leaflets of the mitral valve in systole with prolapse of the posterior leaflet into the left atrium.

17

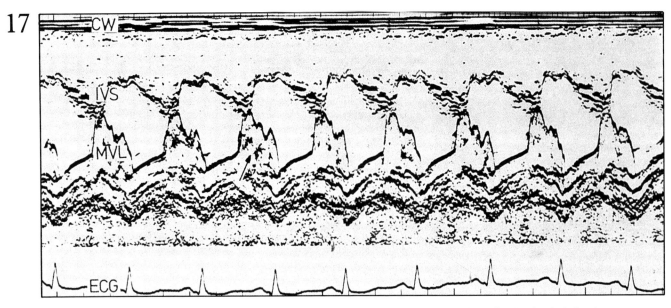

M-mode echocardiogram showing echoes (arrowed) arising from vegetations on the mitral valve in infective endocarditis.

18

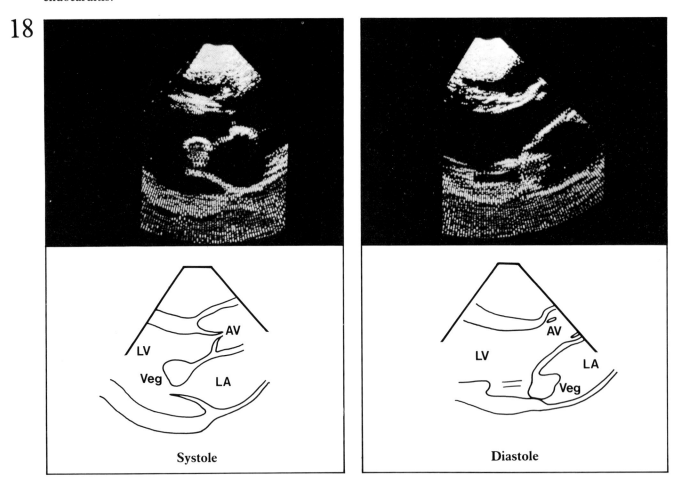

2-D echocardiographic parasternal long axis views of a vegetation attached to the mitral valve leaflet.

19

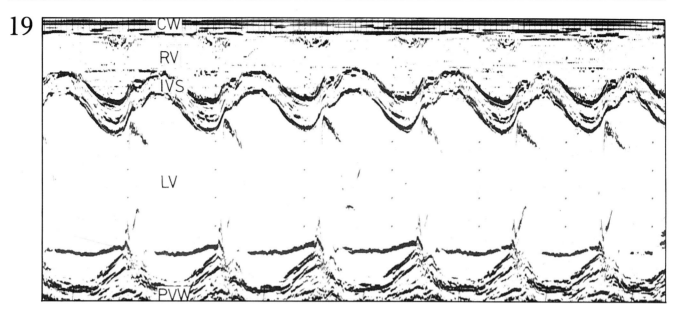

M-mode echocardiogram showing increased end-systolic and end-diastolic dimensions of the left ventricle in pure mitral regurgitation. Ejection fraction is normal.

20

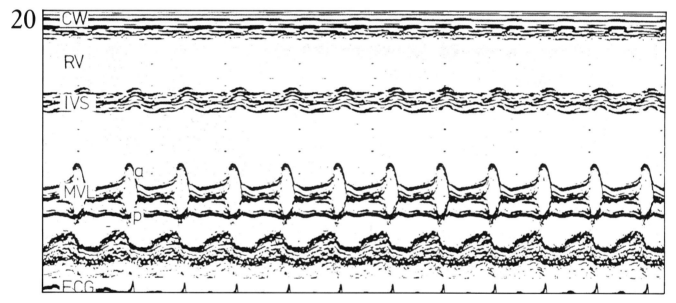

M-mode echocardiogram in dilated cardiomyopathy with secondary mitral regurgitation. Left ventricular dimensions are increased in systole and diastole, but the ejection fraction is reduced.

21

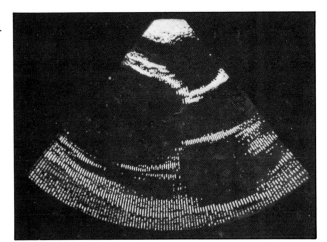
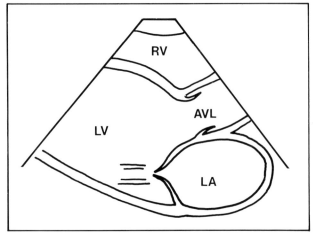

2-D echocardiographic parasternal long axis view showing left ventricular dilatation in a case of dilated cardiomyopathy. Note the thin-walled globular shape of the left ventricle. The left atrium is also enlarged.

22 A prominent 'V' wave is recorded in the pulmonary capillary wedge pressure in a patient with mitral regurgitation.

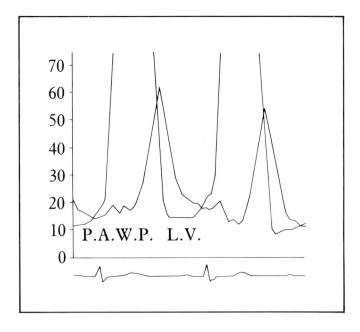

23 Left ventricular angiogram (antero-posterior projection) showing a ballooned posterior mitral leaflet.

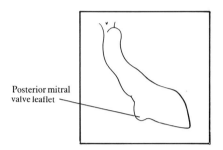

Posterior mitral
valve leaflet

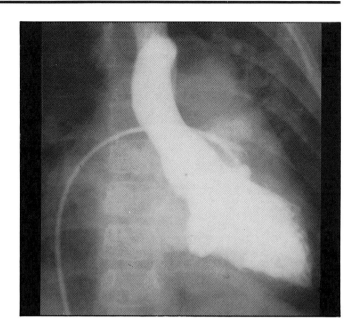

Fixed obstruction to left ventricular outflow can occur at 3 levels. Most frequently it is at valve level (aortic valve stenosis), but it may also be found above or beneath the valve (supravalvular aortic stenosis and subvalvular aortic stenosis respectively). This section deals with these 3 conditions; muscular, dynamic outflow tract obstruction which forms part of the spectrum of hypertrophic cardiomyopathy is considered elsewhere.

Pathology

Aortic Valve Stenosis

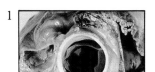
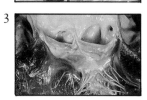
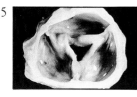
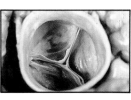
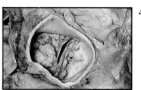
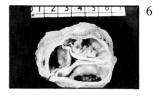
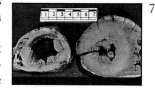

The normal aortic valve is tricuspid [1,2]. The commonest cause of isolated aortic stenosis in the adult is a congenitally bicuspid valve [3]. Dystrophic calcification of the biscupid valve only develops with time and is rarely present before the age of 45 [4]. Up to 1% of the population are born with bicuspid aortic valves, but in only a proportion of these will the valve calcify and produce stenosis.

Rheumatic aortic stenosis is characterized by fusion of all 3 commissures to produce a central triangular aperture [5]. In the majority of these patients, co-existent mitral valve disease is also present.

Senile calcific aortic stenosis occurs as a result of dystrophic calcification in the normal tricuspid aortic valve [6]. It is essentially an accelerated or exaggerated ageing change and is unusual below 65 years of age.

Mixed forms of aortic valve stenosis also occur. Patients with bicuspid valves may develop rheumatic disease resulting in commissural fusion or infective endocarditis which usually produces aortic regurgitation. Dystrophic calcification may also occur in mildly affected rheumatic aortic valves.

All forms of aortic valve stenosis cause obstruction to left ventricular outflow and therefore produce left ventricular hypertrophy characterized by a small cavity and thick wall [7]. In the end-stage, considerable subendocardial fibrosis may occur leading to papillary muscle dysfunction and a dilated left ventricular cavity.

Supravalvular Aortic Stenosis

Supravalvular aortic stenosis occurs as a fibrous shelf or diaphragm across the aortic root above the aortic valve. The lesion is congenital and may be associated with hypercalcaemia and a characteristic facies.

Subvalvular Aortic Stenosis

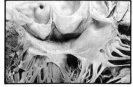

In fixed subvalvular aortic stenosis, the obstruction lies immediately below the aortic valve in the left ventricular outflow tract. The obstruction to outflow has diaphragmatic and fibromuscular components. The diaphragmatic portion, which is attached to the anterior leaflet of the mitral valve, consists of cusp-like tissue and extends forward to insert just below the right coronary cusp of the aortic valve [8]. The fibromuscular component protrudes anteriorly from the ventricular septum opposite the anterior mitral cusp. Cases of fixed subvalvular aortic stenosis may develop muscular hypertrophy causing the septum to bulge.

Presentation

In childhood, patients with asymptomatic aortic stenosis may present at a routine clinical examination during which a cardiac murmur is heard. Furthermore, even in later life certain patients with severe aortic stenosis may remain symptom free.

Symptoms

Some patients with severe aortic stenosis suffer from angina pectoris. Various factors may contribute to the development of this symptom: the hypertrophied left ventricle requires an increased coronary blood flow which is not met, or patients with aortic stenosis may have co-existing coronary artery disease. Exertional syncope may occur as a result of impaired cerebral perfusion due either to relatively fixed cardiac output on exercise or to transient ventricular arrhythmias. Exertional dyspnoea may also be a presenting symptom.

Signs

Fixed obstruction to left ventricular outflow due either to aortic valve stenosis or subvalvular aortic stenosis results in a slow rise of the aortic pressure pulse which can be detected clinically as a slow rise in the cartoid pulse. In supravalvular aortic stenosis, the arterial pulses in the neck are asymmetrical with usually the right carotid having a sharp upstroke while the left is slow-rising due to preferential propagation of the high velocity jet into the innominate artery. Turbulence created at the site of obstruction to left ventricular outflow gives rise to an ejection systolic murmur.

In aortic valve stenosis the abrupt halting of the abnormal domed valve gives rise to an aortic ejection sound which is not a feature of subvalvular or supravalvular aortic stenosis. Obstruction to left ventricular outflow results in prolongation of left ventricular ejection. This causes a delay in closure of the aortic valve and, consequently, reversed splitting of the second heart sound may be heard. If the obstruction is due to valvular aortic stenosis and the valve is rigid and immobile, then neither the ejection sound nor the aortic component of the second heart sound may be heard.

The hypertrophied stiff left ventricle gives rise to two abnormal palpatory findings. The apical impulse is usually sustained in quality during systole, but is not markedly exaggerated. In addition, the abnormally powerful left atrial contraction can be palpated as a separate atrial (double) impulse and may be audible as a fourth heart sound.

Investigations

Radiology

Valvular Aortic Stenosis

In uncomplicated aortic valve stenosis, the heart size remains

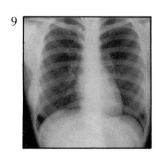

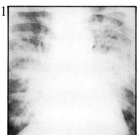

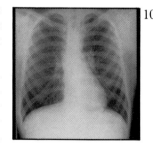

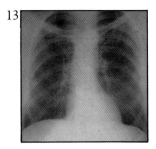

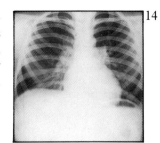

within normal limits [9], but the ascending aorta shows post-stenotic dilatation [10]. Although all cases of severe aortic stenosis develop left ventricular hypertrophy, in the later stages dilatation of the left ventricle may also occur leading to left ventricular failure [11]. The aortic cusps become irregular, disorganized and calcified [12].

Supravalvular and Subvalvular Aortic Stenosis

In supravalvular aortic stenosis the chest radiograph shows a normal sized heart with an inconspicuous aorta [13]. There may also be evidence of associated pulmonary artery stenoses [14].

In subvalvular aortic stenosis the chest radiograph is usually normal, although occasionally post-stenotic dilatation of the aorta may be present.

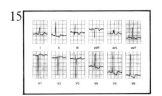

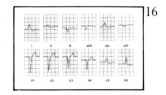

Electrocardiography

The electrocardiogram may remain normal even in severe left ventricular outflow obstruction, but it is more usual for it to reflect left ventricular hypertrophy with ST-segment and T-wave abnormalities in the left ventricular leads [15]. Left bundle branch block may also be seen [16].

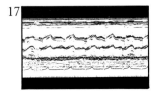

Echocardiography

Valvular Aortic Stenosis

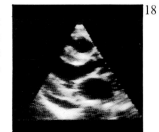

Although it may appear normal, the M-mode echocardiogram of a bicuspid non-calcified aortic valve typically has an eccentric diastolic closure line; almost invariably it is displaced anteriorly [17]. The bicuspid valve usually domes during systole [18]. In calcified aortic stenosis, dense parallel echoes are seen in the aortic root due to multiple re-reflection of the ultrasound beam at the interfaces of the calcific material. In mild cases, it is still possible to visualize some cusp movement or at least to appreciate clearing of the echoes as the calcified leaflets separate in systole [19], but, as the pathological process progresses, the echoes obliterate the space of the aortic root and are present throughout the cardiac cycle [20].

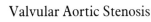

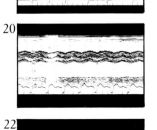

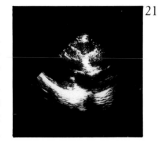

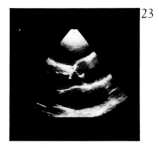

It is usually easier to visualize the aortic valve and its abnormal structure and movement by 2-dimensional echocardiography than from M-mode recordings [21].

Supravalvular and Subvalvular Aortic Stenosis

The region of narrowing in supravalvular aortic stenosis may be demonstrated echocardiographically by scanning upwards from the aortic root [22]. If a definite increase in diameter is seen, this provides strong evidence of a reduction in aortic size.

It is often possible to visualize the obstruction in subvalvular aortic stenosis in the long axis view [23]. Occasionally, M-mode echocardiography shows that the aortic valve leaflets close progressively throughout systole with a coarse fluttering motion indistinguishable from that seen in hypertrophic cardiomyopathy. Subvalvular aortic stenosis is commonly associated with minor

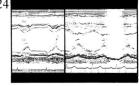

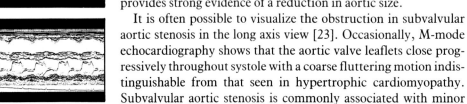

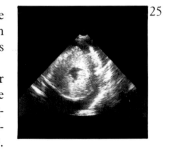

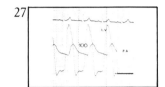

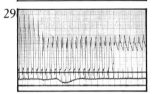

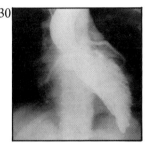

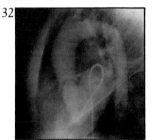

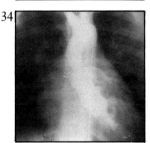

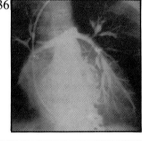

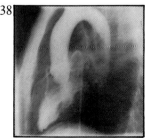

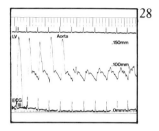

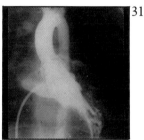

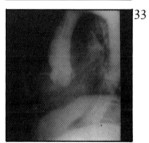

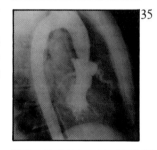

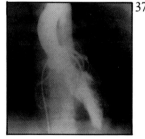

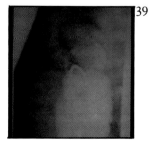

valvular incompetence which is detected by the fluttering of the anterior mitral valve cusp in diastole.

In fixed left ventricular outflow obstruction, the left ventricle is usually symmetrically hypertrophied and this is reflected echocardiographically as an increased thickness of both the septum and posterior wall and a reduction in ventricular diameter [24,25]. Although the hypertrophy is usually symmetrical, the septum may be thicker than the free wall as in cases of hypertrophic cardiomyopathy. On M-mode echocardiography, the anterior mitral valve leaflet may show a decreased diastolic closure rate in severe left ventricular hypertrophy from any cause [26] and it is important to distinguish this appearance from rheumatic mitral stenosis by demonstration of the normal opposite movement of the posterior cusp or by 2-dimensional echocardiography.

Cardiac Catheterization and Angiography

In valvular aortic stenosis, there is a systolic pressure difference across the valve [27] while in supravalvular stenosis the pressure difference is between the supravalvular chamber and the aorta [28] and in subvalvular aortic stenosis it is within the left ventricle [29].

Left ventricular hypertrophy may be seen by left ventriculography [30]. In valvular aortic stenosis the typical change is the thickening of the cusps, with doming in systole, and a central ejection jet may be seen [31,32,33].

In supravalvular stenosis, angiography shows the obstructive lesion above the sinuses of Valsalva [34,35]. If additional pulmonary artery stenoses are present, they may be seen on right ventricular angiograms [36].

In subvalvular aortic stenosis, the left ventricular angiogram shows the subvalvular obstruction [37,38] or a more diffuse fibromuscular lesion [39]. Associated aortic valve regurgitation may be demonstrated by aortography.

1 Fully open normal aortic valve. The cusps fold back into the aortic sinuses to leave a large central opening.

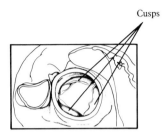

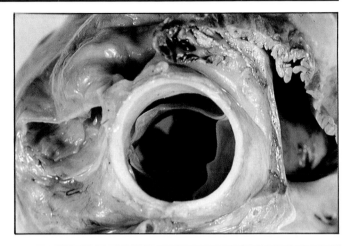

2 Fully closed normal aortic valve. The cusps meet and overlap providing support for each other in the closed position.

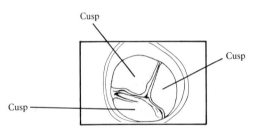

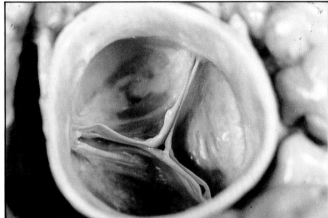

3 A bicuspid aortic valve. The opened valve has only two cusps which at this age have not undergone calcification.

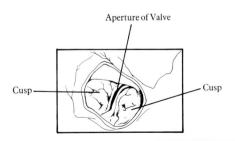

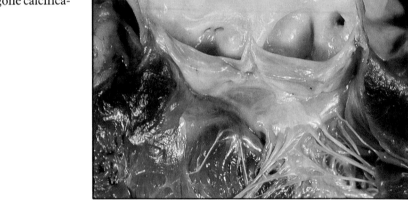

4 Calcific bicuspid aortic stenosis. The aperture of the valve is a transverse slit across the aortic root between two cusps. Masses of calcium bulge from each cusp.

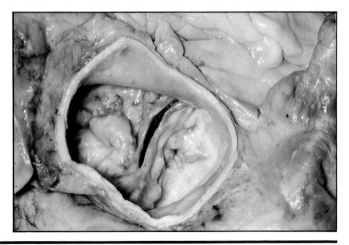

5 Rheumatic aortic stenosis in a patient with co-existent mitral disease. The aortic valve aperture is triangular due to fusion of all three commissures.

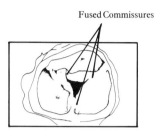

Fused Commissures

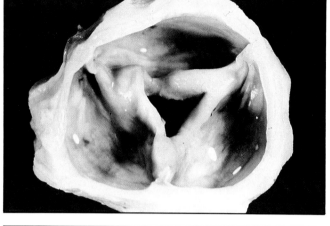

6 Pure 'senile' aortic stenosis in a tricuspid aortic valve due to extreme age-related dystrophic calcification in the cusps.

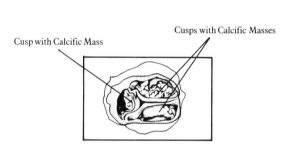

Cusp with Calcific Mass   Cusps with Calcific Masses

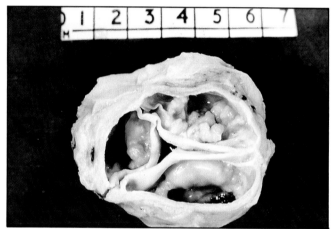

7 Transverse slice of left ventricle from a patient with a normal heart compared with a patient with aortic stenosis. In aortic stenosis the ventricular wall is thick and the cavity is small.

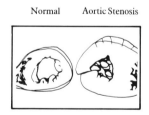

Normal   Aortic Stenosis

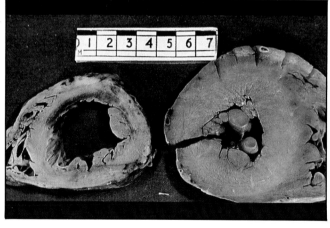

8 The aortic outflow tract in a case with subvalvular aortic stenosis. A membrane joins the anterior cusp of the mitral valve to the interventricular septum beneath the aortic valve.

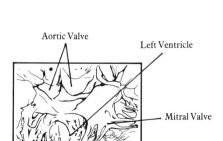

Aortic Valve   Left Ventricle

Mitral Valve

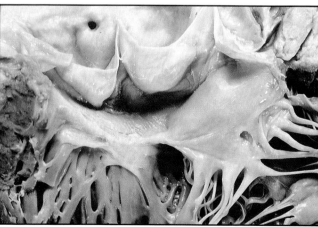

9 Chest radiograph of uncomplicated aortic valve stenosis, showing normal heart size.

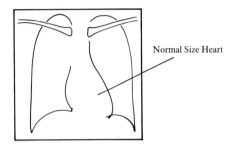

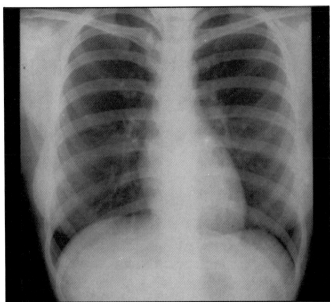

10 Chest radiograph of aortic valve stenosis showing post-stenotic dilatation of the ascending aorta.

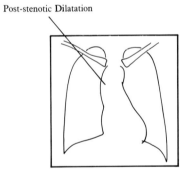

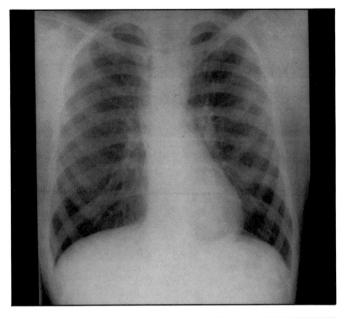

11 Chest radiograph of aortic valve stenosis in left ventricular failure showing pulmonary oedema.

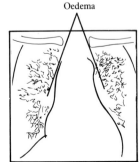

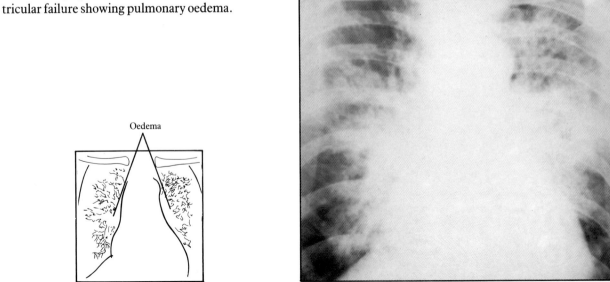

12 Chest radiograph (lateral projection) in aortic valve stenosis showing a calcified aortic valve.

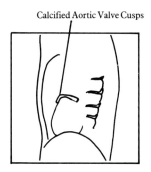

Calcified Aortic Valve Cusps

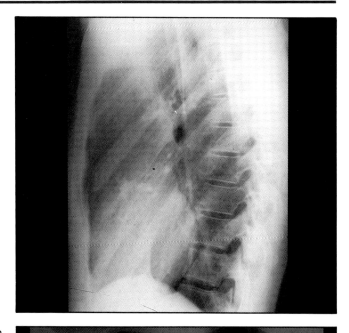

13 Chest radiograph in supravalvular aortic stenosis. The heart size is normal and the ascending aorta inconspicuous.

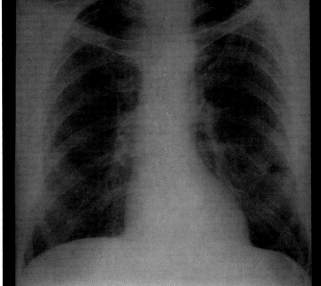

Aorta

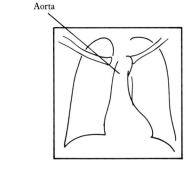

14 Chest radiograph in supravalvular aortic stenosis associated with central pulmonary artery stenosis. The aortic arch is inconspicuous; there is post-stenotic dilatation of the pulmonary arteries.

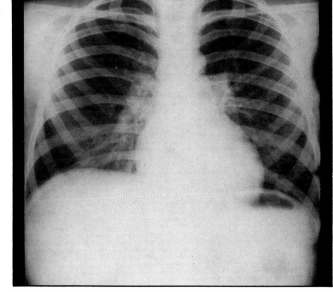

Post-stenotic Dilatation

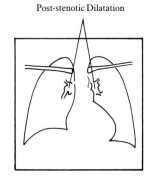

15

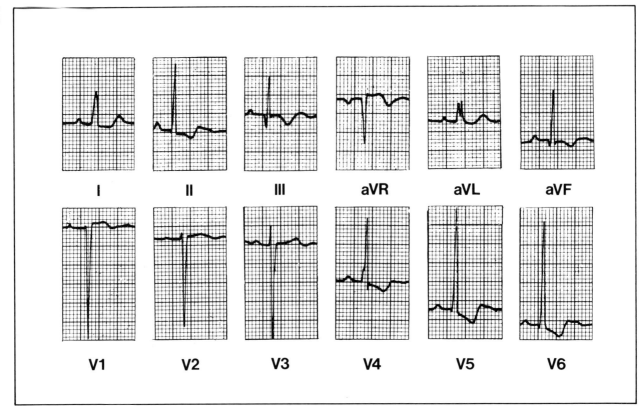

Electrocardiogram in severe aortic stenosis showing deep S wave in V1 and tall R wave in V5 with ST and T-wave changes indicating left ventricular hypertrophy.

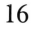**16**

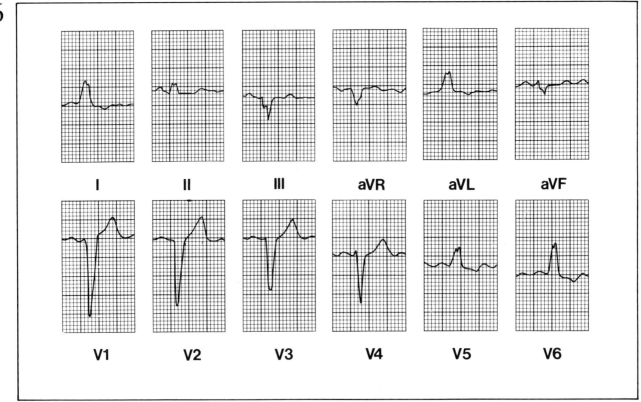

Electrocardiogram in a patient with aortic stenosis showing left bundle branch block.

17

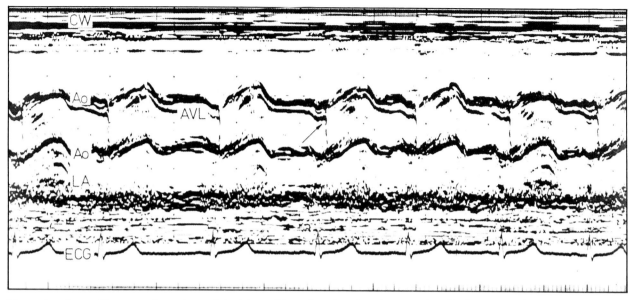

M-mode echocardiogram of a patient with a bicuspid aortic valve showing anterior displacement of the diastolic closure line (arrowed).

18

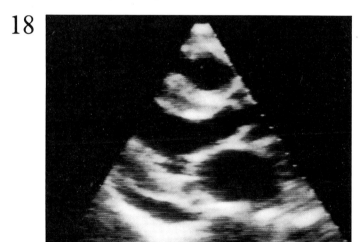 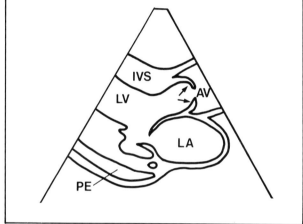

2-D parasternal long axis echocardiographic view showing doming of the aortic valve leaflets in systole (arrows). A pericardial effusion is also present.

19

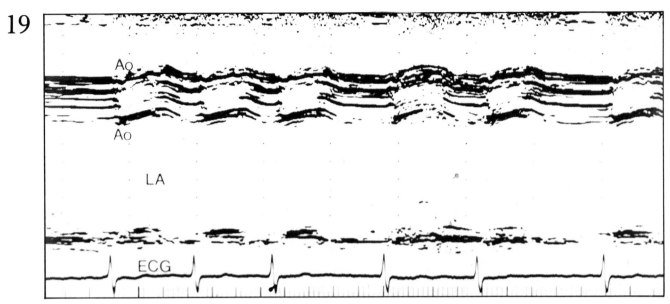

M-mode echocardiogram in calcific aortic stenosis showing multiple echoes in the aortic root which partially clear during systole.

20

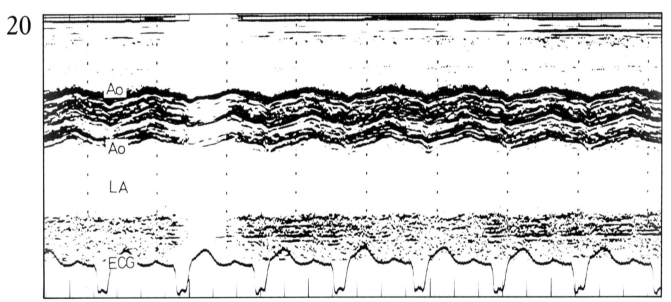

M-mode echocardiograms in calcific aortic stenosis showing obliteration of the aortic root by dense echoes through the cardiac cycle.

21

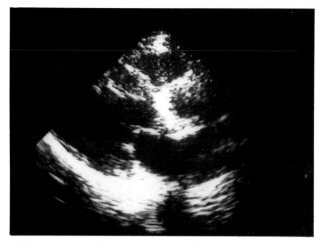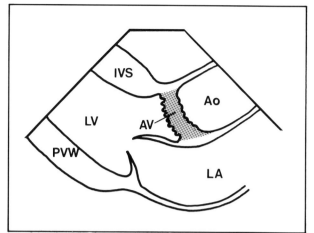

2-D parasternal long axis echocardiographic view showing a thickened calcified aortic valve.

22

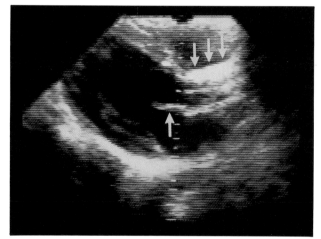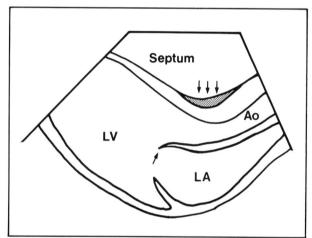

2-D echocardiographic parasternal long axis view showing supravalvular aortic stenosis (arrowed).

23

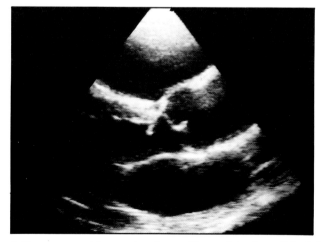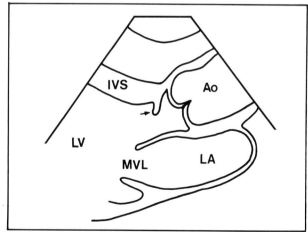

2-D parasternal long axis echocardiographic view of the left ventricle and outflow tract showing discrete subaortic membrane obstructing the outflow tract (arrowed).

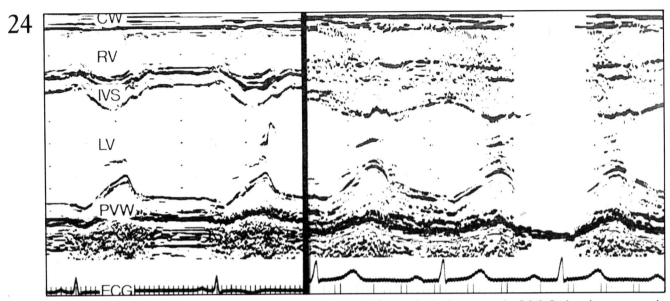

M-mode echocardiogram of a normal left ventricle [left], and left ventricular hypertrophy [right], showing symmetrical thickening of the septum and left ventricular posterior wall and reduction of cavity size.

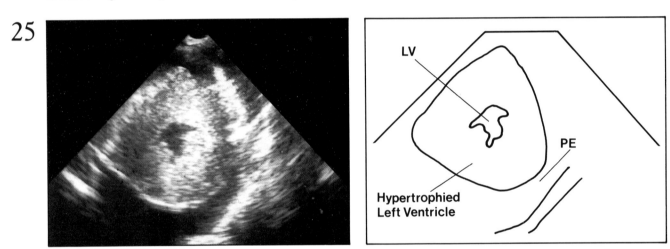

2-D short axis echocardiographic view showing concentric hypertrophy of the left ventricle with a small left ventricular cavity. There is an additional pericardial effusion.

26

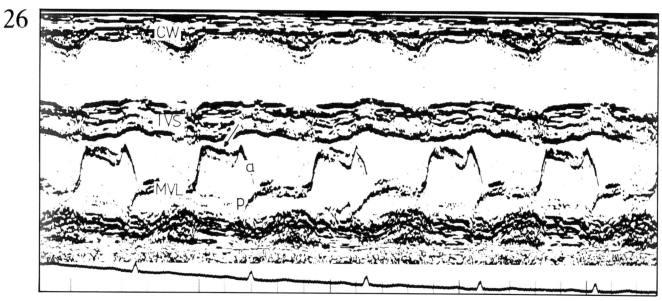

M-mode echocardiogram in aortic stenosis showing reduction in diastolic closure rate of the anterior leaflet of the mitral valve (arrow), but normal posterior cusp movement indicating a normal mitral valve.

27

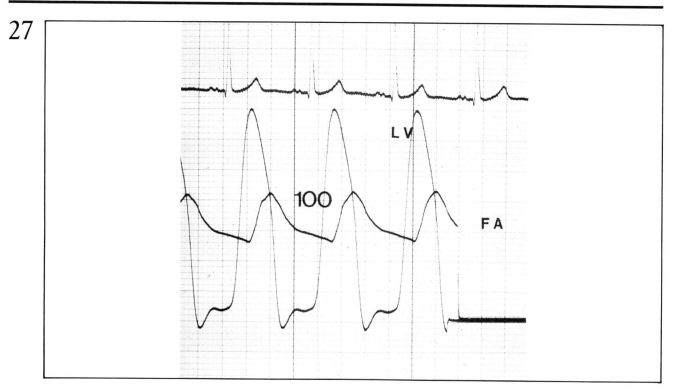

Pressure tracing showing gradient across the aortic valve.

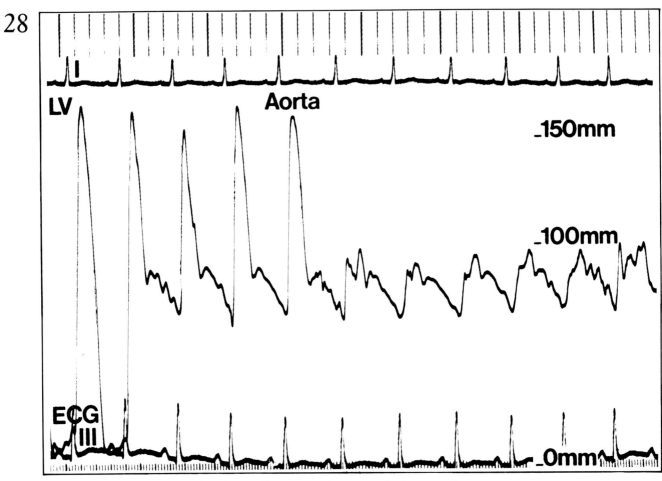

Withdrawal pressure tracing showing gradient across the supravalvular stenosis.

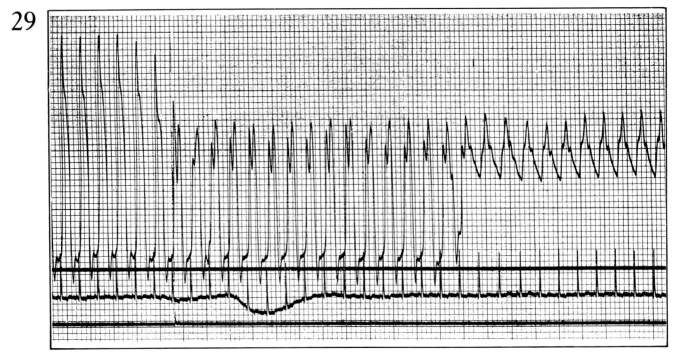

Withdrawal pressure tracing showing gradient across a subvalvular stenosis.

30 Left ventricular angiogram (right anterior oblique projection) in aortic valve stenosis showing gross left ventricular hypertrophy.

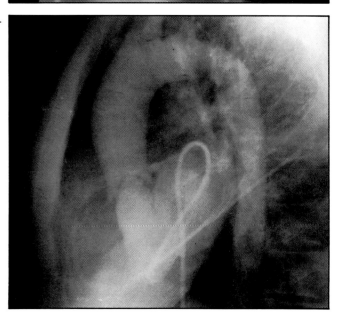

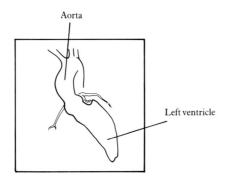

Aorta

Left ventricle

31 Systolic frame from the same patient as [30] showing a thick domed valve.

Thick Domed Aortic Cusps

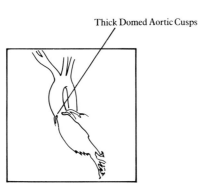

32 Lateral view of a ventricular angiogram in aortic stenosis showing a thick domed valve with post-stenotic dilatation of the aorta.

Thick Aortic Valve Cusps

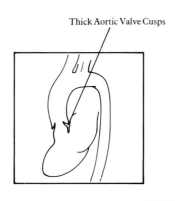

33 Lateral view of an aortogram in aortic stenosis, showing thick irregular rigid cusps of the aortic valve.

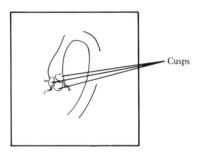

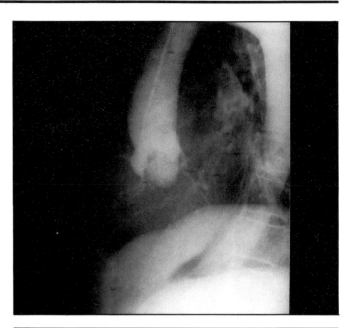

34 Left ventricular angiogram (antero-posterior projection) showing supravalvular stenosis and left ventricular hypertrophy.

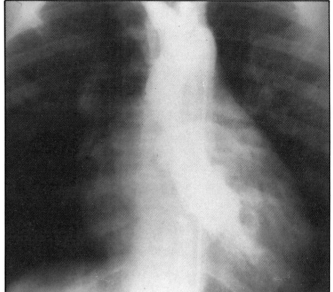

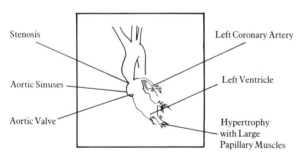

35 Lateral view of [34].

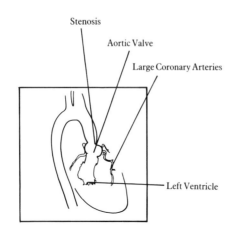

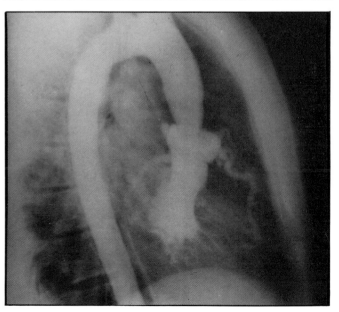

36 Right ventricular angiogram (antero posterior projection) in the same patient as [34,35] showing pulmonary artery stenosis.

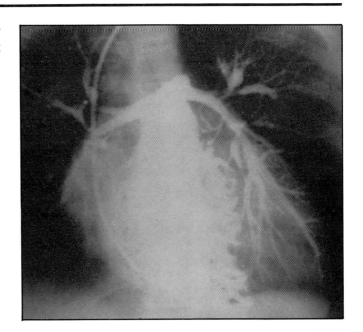

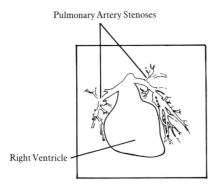

37 Left ventricular angiogram (antero-posterior projection) showing diaphragmatic subvalvular aortic stenosis and left ventricular hypertrophy.

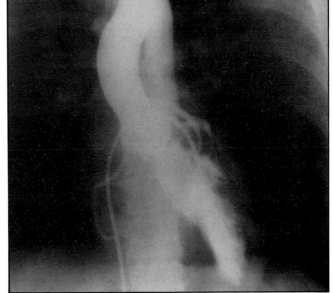

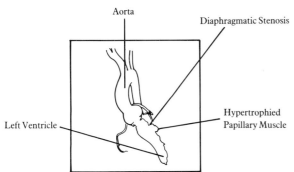

38 Lateral view of [37].

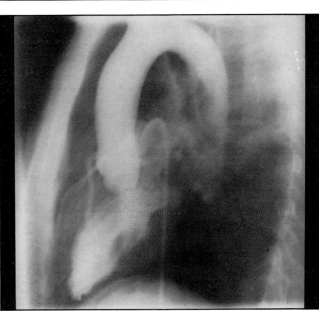

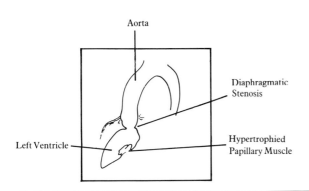

39 Left ventricular angiogram (lateral projection) with tunnel subvalvular aortic stenosis.

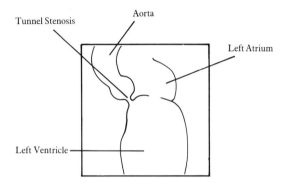

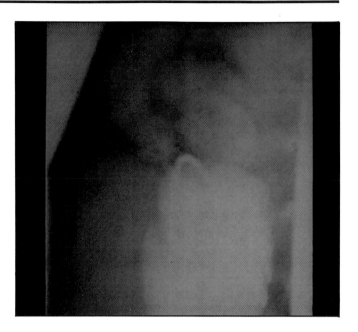

AORTIC REGURGITATION

Pathology

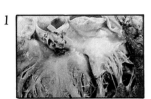

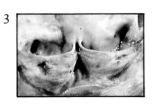

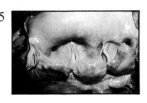

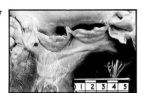

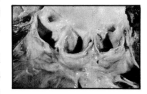

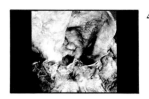

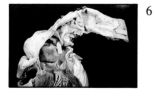

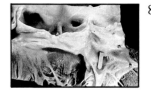

Aortic regurgitation results either from disease of the aortic cusps or disease of the aortic wall leading to aortic root dilatation. Infective endocarditis involving either the bicuspid or tricuspid aortic valve may result in perforation of a cusp and consequent aortic regurgitation [1]. Other causes of aortic regurgitation due to cusp disease include a chronic rheumatic process [2] and even rheumatoid granulomata.

Aortic root dilatation occurs in both inflammatory aortitis and medial aortic degeneration. The causes of aortitis include syphilis [3] and ankylosing spondylitis [4]. Syphilis produces characteristic widening, i.e. separation of the cusp edges at the commissures. Ankylosing spondylitis in contrast produces a more distorted aortic root but commissure widening is less marked. In all forms of aortitis the intima is often wrinkled and scarred (tree barking) expressing underlying medial destruction. Distinction of the various types of aortitis without serology and clinical history is usually impossible, as the histology is uniform. Aortic medial degeneration is characterized by loss of muscle and elastic tissue in the aortic root. In some instances focal accumulation of acid mucopolysaccharide is found. Such changes occur in Marfan's syndrome [5 & 6]. It is more common for these changes to be an isolated finding without other skeletal stigmata of Marfan's syndrome than to have a greater degree of mucin accumulation in the media (cystic medial necrosis).

Chronic aortic regurgitation leads to left ventricular dilatation often with associated hypertrophy. Regurgitant jets across the valve may hit the interventricular septum [7] or the ventricular aspect of the anterior cusp of the mitral valve [8] producing patches of endocardial thickening.

Presentation

Symptoms

Patients with slight aortic regurgitation may present following the finding of a cardiac murmur at routine medical examination. Symptoms are rare in chronic aortic regurgitation unless the lesion is severe. Patients who complain of exertional dyspnoea, or dyspnoea at rest, do so because the pulmonary venous pressure is raised - a change which occurs late in the natural history of the disease. Angina occurs occasionally in patients with aortic regurgitation. This may be the result of aortitis affecting the origin of the coronary arteries, or because of coronary atheroma. Angina can also occur without coronary artery narrowing because coronary perfusion is inadequate to meet the demands of the enlarged left ventricle.

In contrast severe aortic regurgitation developing acutely (due to aortic dissection) or over a short period (as in infective endocarditis) is poorly tolerated. Pulmonary oedema in these circumstances develops rapidly because there is a rapid increase in left ventricular diastolic pressure (and hence pulmonary venous pressure) in the presence of a previously normal left ventricle.

Signs

The constant physical sign of aortic regurgitation is the presence of an early diastolic murmur. This may be accompanied by a systolic murmur due to increased stroke volume through a normal aortic valve or one with abnormal leaflets. The presence of an ejection sound may be associated either with a bicuspid aortic valve or with aortic root dilatation. In slight aortic regurgitation there will be no other abnormality. In moderate or severe chronic aortic regurgitation there will be a wide pulse pressure with a rapid upstroke and downstroke in the arterial pulses. The apical impulse will be hyperdynamic reflecting the large stroke volume of the left ventricle. A mid-diastolic murmur may be heard in the mitral area (Austin-Flint murmur). In acute severe aortic regurgitation the clinical picture will be dominated by pulmonary oedema.

Investigations

Radiology

If aortic regurgitation is due to abnormalities of the aortic wall then the ascending aorta on the chest x-ray may be seen to be enlarged. Usually there is generalised dilatation of the ascending aorta [9], but in syphilis a localised aneurysm may be seen [10]. If aortic regurgitation is due to a leaflet abnormality, the ascending aorta may appear normal.

In long standing aortic regurgitation, the left ventricle dilates producing cardiac enlargement in the chest x-ray [11]. In acute aortic regurgitation as from perforation of a cusp there may be pulmonary oedema but the cardiac silhouette remains normal [12].

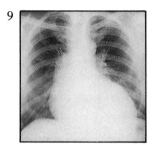

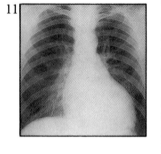

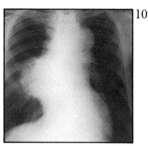

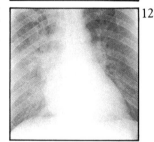

Electrocardiography

The electrocardiogram usually reflects left ventricular enlargement. Large voltages may be present in V1 (deep S wave) and V5 (tall R wave) [13]. There may be associated ST-T changes [14]. In acute aortic regurgitation the electrocardiogram may be normal even though the aortic regurgitation may be severe.

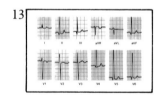

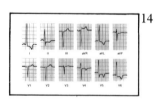

Echocardiography

In aortic wall disease the aortic valve leaflets are usually normal. However, dilatation of the aorta may be detected by echocardiography [15,16,17]. In aortic regurgitation due to acute dissection of the aortic root it is frequently possible to visualize the intra mural separation [18]. Most patients with dissection extending back to the aortic root have an increased amount of pericardial fluid which is readily detected by echocardiography.

Where aortic regurgitation is due to a leaflet abnormality, such as prolapse of the leaflet, calcification or a vegetation, it may be visualized directly [19,20].

Dilatation of the left ventricle occurs as a consequence of moderate or severe aortic regurgitation and can be detected echocardiographically [21]. The severity of chronic aortic regurgita-

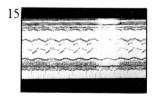

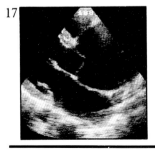

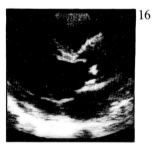

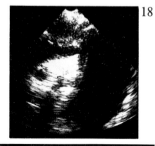

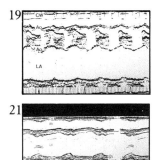

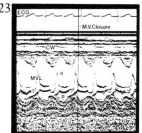

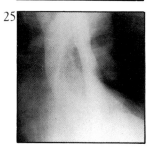

tion can be assessed by calculation of the left ventricular stroke volume. It is possible to estimate left ventricular stroke volume from the echocardiogram by reference to end-diastolic and end-systolic dimensions. Calculated fractional shortening remains normal until left ventricular failure supervenes.

The regurgitant jet of blood impinging on the anterior mitral valve leaflet causes fluttering in diastole [22]. This sign is not related to the severity of the regurgitation but is a very sensitive method of detecting aortic regurgitation. Sometimes the jet is directed at the septal endocardium and this may then be seen to flutter.

In acute severe aortic regurgitation (as occurs in endocarditis) premature closure of the mitral valve detected echocardiographically indicates severe haemodynamic disturbance [23]. However left ventricular dimensions may remain close to normal.

Cardiac Catheterization and Angiography

Elevation of the left ventricular end-diastolic pressure is often present in patients with moderate or severe aortic regurgitation. The highest end-diastolic pressures are seen in patients with acute severe aortic regurgitation and this may exceed left atrial pressure causing premature closure of the mitral valve.

Aortic regurgitation can be demonstrated by aortography which also demonstrates the anatomy of the aortic root [24]. An ascending aortogram is the best method of diagnosing dissection of the aorta [25].

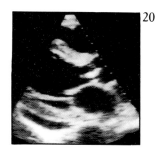

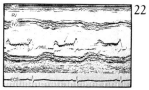

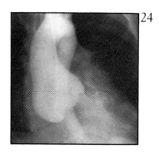

1   Infective endocarditis of the aortic valve with perforation of a cusp (arrowed) producing incompetence. Vegetation present on the valve.

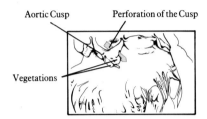

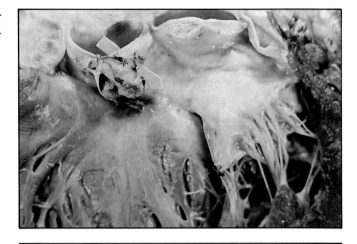

2   Rheumatic aortic incompetence: all three cusps are fibrotic and retracted. Note the coexistent thickening of mitral chordae.

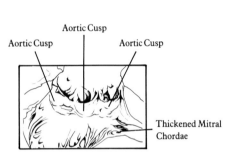

3   Mild syphilitic aortic valve disease. The commissure is widened, the two cusps not meeting. The ascending aorta shows pearly yellow flat plaques.

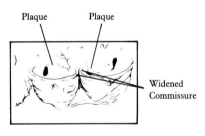

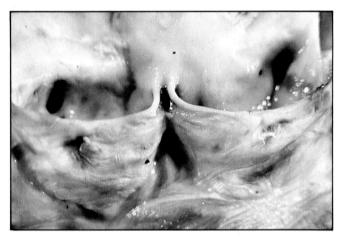

4   Ankylosing spondylitis with aortic regurgitation. The aortic root is dilated, the intima wrinkled; the valve cusps are distorted and shrunken.

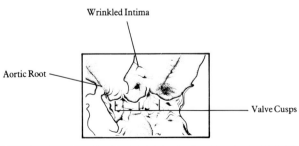

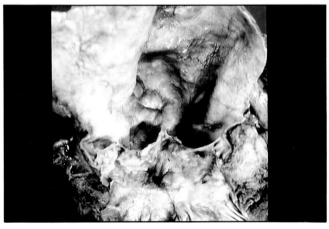

5 Dilated aortic root with ballooned thin aortic cusps producing aortic incompetence in Marfan's syndrome.

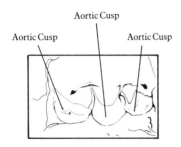

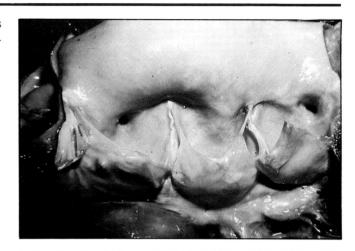

6 Aorta in Marfan's syndrome. The aortic root is dilated and there are two healed dissection tears (arrowed).

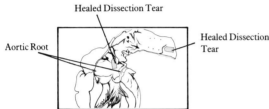

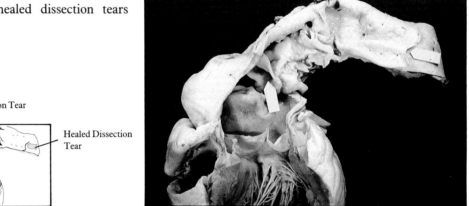

7 Aortic root dilatation with a patch of endocardial thickening on the ventricular septum due to impingement of a regurgitant jet.

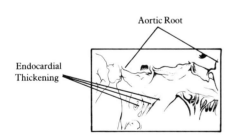

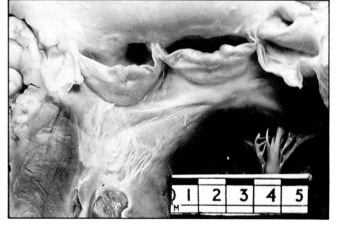

8 Biscupid aortic valve with a cleft in the largest cusp producing mild aortic regurgitation. Jet lesion on the ventricular surface of the anterior cusp of the mitral valve (arrow).

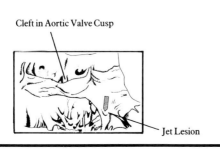

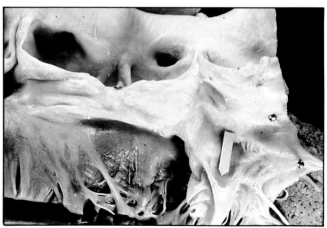

AORTIC REGURGITATION Radiology

9 Chest radiograph showing dilatation of the ascending aorta due to Marfan's syndrome with cardiac enlargement from resultant aortic regurgitation.

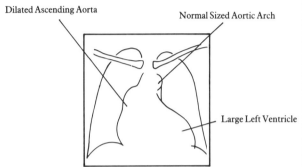
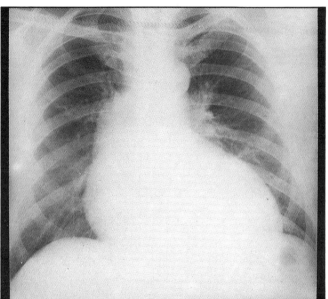

10 Chest radiograph showing a localized aneurysm of the ascending aorta due to syphilis.

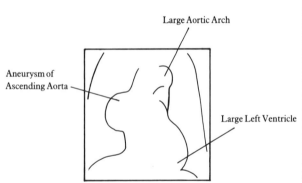
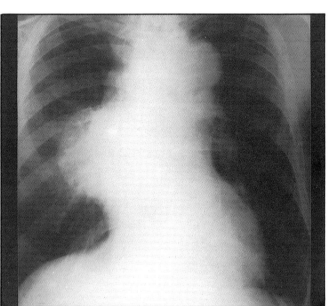

11 Chest radiograph showing cardiac enlargement in chronic aortic regurgitation.

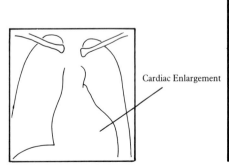
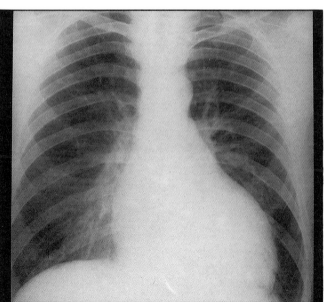

12 Chest radiograph showing pulmonary oedema with normal heart size due to acute aortic regurgitation from a ruptured cusp.

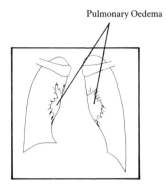

Pulmonary Oedema

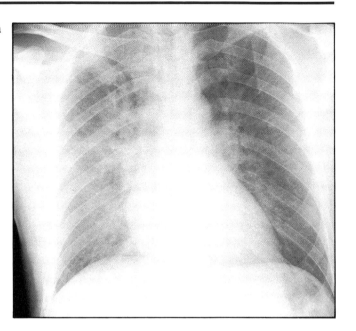

AORTIC REGURGITATION

Electrocardiography

13

| I | II | III | aVR | aVL | aVF |

| V1 | V2 | V3 | V4 | V5 | V6 |

The electrocardiogram in chronic aortic regurgitation showing increased left ventricular voltage (deep S wave V1, tall R wave V6).

14

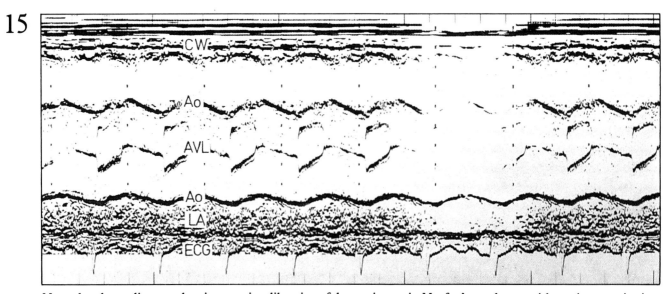

I	II	III	aVR	aVL	aVF
V1	V2	V3	V4	V5	V6

The electrocardiogram in chronic aortic regurgitation showing severe left ventricular hypertrophy (i.e. increased voltage and ST-T wave abnormalities in the lateral leads).

15

CW

Ao

AVL

Ao

LA

ECG

M-mode echocardiogram showing massive dilatation of the aortic root in Marfan's syndrome with aortic regurgitation.

16

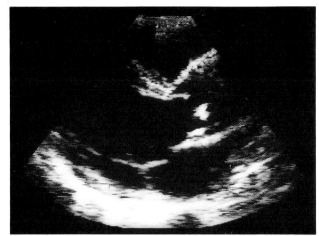 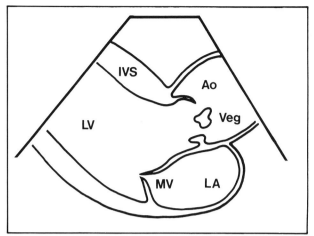

2-D echocardiographic parasternal long axis systolic frame in aortic regurgitation due to infective endocarditis showing the vegetation being carried up the ascending aorta during ejection. The vegetation is attached to the non-coronary aortic cusp. Note the shape of the right coronary cusp suggesting that the valve is bicuspid.

17

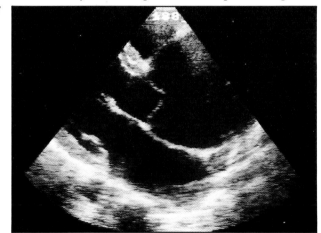 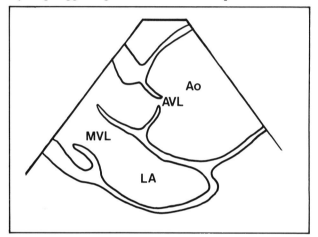

2-D echocardiographic parasternal long axis view in a case of aortic regurgitation secondary to aneurysmal dilatation of the aortic root. This is a diastolic frame, as shown by the wide open mitral valve, yet the aortic cusps fail to appose and one is prolapsing below the other.

18

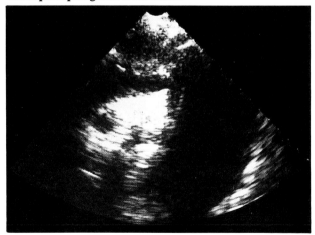 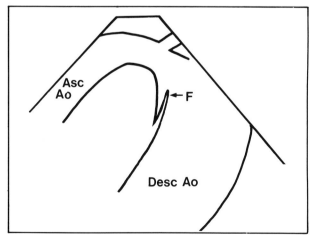

2-D echocardiographic suprasternal long axis view of the aortic arch showing the intimal flap in a patient with Marfan's syndrome and aortic dissection.

19

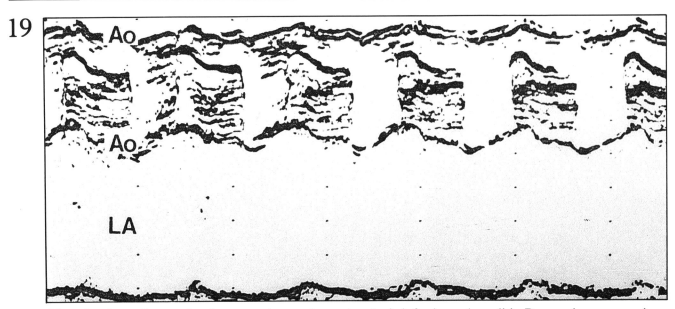

M-mode echocardiogram showing vegetations on the aortic valve in infective endocarditis. Dense echoes are seen in diastole with clearing in systole.

20

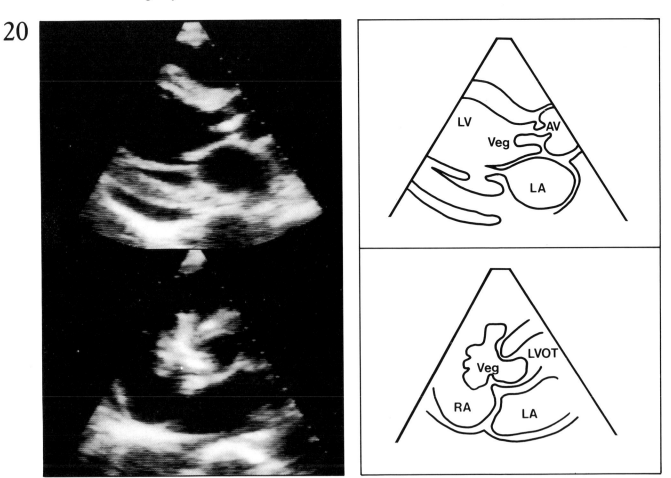

2-D echocardiographic views of aortic vegetations. Above, parasternal long axis view showing vegetations prolapsing into the left ventricular outflow tract. Below, modified parasternal short axis view of the aortic root showing the aortic vegetation invading across the aortic wall to the tricuspid valve.

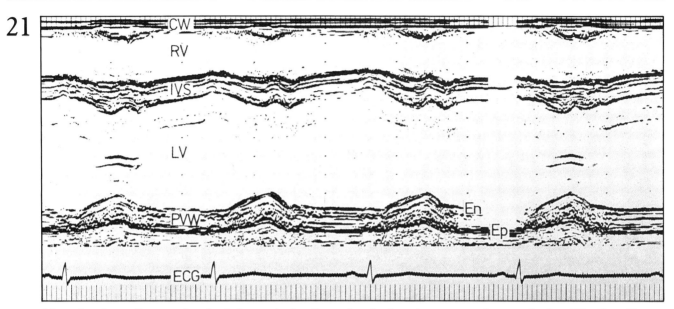

M-mode echocardiogram showing left ventricular dimensions in chronic severe aortic regurgitation. The diastolic diameter is greatly increased (6.4 cms) but fractional shortening is normal.

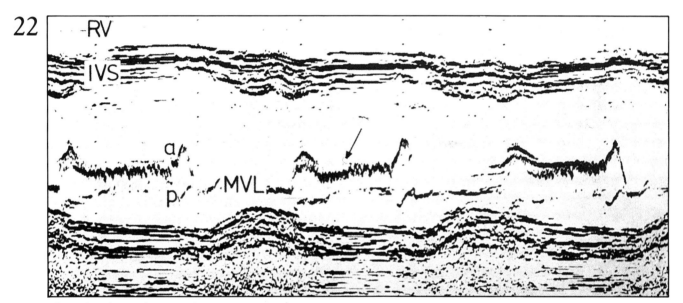

M-mode echocardiogram of the mitral valve in aortic regurgitation showing fluttering of its anterior leaflet in diastole (arrowed).

23 M-mode echocardiogram showing premature closure of the mitral valve in acute severe aortic regurgitation.

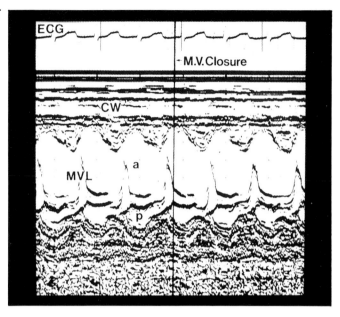

24 Aortogram (antero-posterior projection) showing aortic root dilatation in Marfan's syndrome.

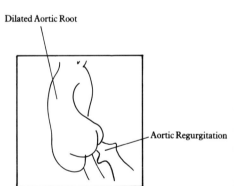

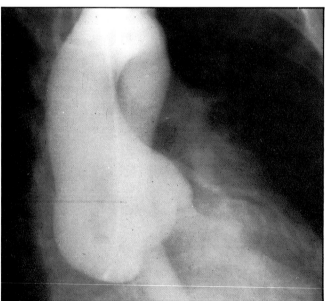

25 Aortogram (antero-posterior projection) of aortic dissection. The true lumen is compressed by the non-opaque false lumen.

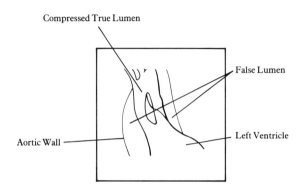

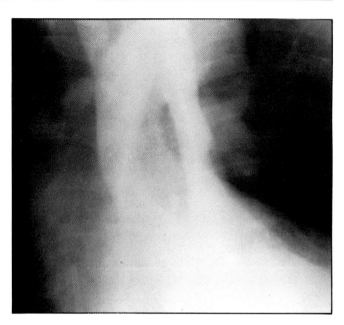

Although there are several congenital malformations that may involve the tricuspid valve (e.g. tricuspid atresia) only Ebstein's anomaly, and acquired tricuspid valve disease, will be considered here.

Pathology

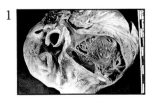

In Ebstein's anomaly the tricuspid valve is patent. In its most severe form, the valve orifice is displaced into the right ventricle down to the junction of the inlet and outlet portions [1]. The valve leaflets are dysplastic and the inlet portion of the ventricle becomes considerably thinned (atrialization).

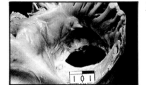

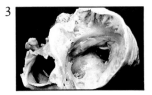

Acquired tricuspid valve disease is unusual. A small proportion of patients with chronic rheumatic valve disease develop involvement of the tricuspid valve in addition to aortic and mitral disease. This produces fusion of the commissures in a manner analogous to mitral valve disease [2]. Acute infective endocarditis of the tricuspid valve is a complication in drug addicts who use intravenous injections. Carcinoid tumours may produce large amounts of vaso-active amines resulting in white fibrous thickening of the surfaces of the tricuspid and pulmonary valves [3]. This leads to tricuspid and pulmonary stenosis and incompetence.

Presentation

Symptoms

Paroxysmal supraventricular tachycardia is the usual presenting feature of an adult with Ebstein's anomaly, though some may have no symptoms at all and are detected as a result of a routine chest x-ray.

The average patient with rheumatic tricuspid valvular disease usually presents with symptoms attributable to the co-existence of rheumatic mitral valve disease. Thus, breathlessness on exertion is not due to tricuspid valve disease but due to the associated mitral valve disease. However when tricuspid stenosis is severe the dypsnoea which normally accompanies severe mitral stenosis may be absent. Tricuspid involvement may cause in addition venous distention resulting in hepatic enlargement, ascites and peripheral oedema.

Fatigue resulting from a low fixed cardiac output is a very common symptom in the patient with severe tricuspid valve disease. Isolated tricuspid regurgitation occurs most frequently as a result of infective endocarditis in drug addicts. The presenting features will be those of infective endocarditis. Right atrial thrombosis or endocarditis of the valve may result in pulmonary embolism.

Signs

Most patients with Ebstein's anomaly are cyanosed. The atria and venous pulses are usually normal but prominent systolic waves in the venous pulse may be seen. The first heart sound may be widely split due to delayed tricuspid closure and the second heart sound is also abnormally wide but moves with respiration. An extra sound characteristically occurs after the two components of the second heart sound; in addition there may be the murmur of tricuspid regurgitation.

The most important clinical clue to the diagnosis of tricuspid valve disease is the alteration in the venous pulse. If tricuspid stenosis is dominant and the patient is in sinus rhythm the abnormally powerful right atrial contraction results in a striking increase in the 'a' wave of the venous pulse. Because there is an obstruction to right atrial emptying the rate of fall of the elevated pressure in diastole is reduced giving rise to a slow 'y' descent. By contrast, in dominant or pure tricuspid regurgitation the right atrial pressure in systole reflects the right ventricular systolic pressure with a marked increase in the 'v' or systolic wave of the venous pulse in the neck. The systolic venous expansion may be transmitted to the liver causing a systolic expansile pulsation. The descent of the venous pulse (y) is prominent and rapid. Peripheral oedema and ascites are common findings in severe tricuspid valve disease due to the high venous pressure.

Tricuspid regurgitation results in a pan-systolic murmur usually best heard at the left sternal edge, the intensity of which is increased by inspiration. In pure tricuspid regurgitation a third heart sound will also be heard at the left sternal edge. With tricuspid stenosis there may be an opening snap and a mid-diastolic murmur both best heard at the left sternal edge during inspiration.

Investigations

Radiology

In Ebstein's anomaly the chest radiograph often shows a large globular heart. There may be a bulge on the left heart border due to displacement of the right ventricular outflow tract [4]. The right heart border may also be prominent and there is frequently pulmonary oligaemia [5].

In rheumatic tricuspid valve disease the radiographic features are often dominated by the associated rheumatic involvement of the mitral or aortic valves. In severe tricuspid stenosis the right atrium may be very large [6]. The normal radiographic features of mitral valve disease may be limited by the presence of tricuspid valve disease. Thus, upper lobe pulmonary venous dilatation due to mitral involvement may be less obvious if there is additional severe tricuspid valve disease [7].

Electrocardiography

In Ebstein's anomaly, the typical features include tall P waves and right bundle branch block [8]. In acquired tricuspid valve disease right atrial hypertrophy may be the only electrocardiographic feature [9].

Echocardiography

In Ebstein's anomaly the tricuspid valve is seen to be large and displaced [10]. The abnormal position of the tricuspid valve causes it to be always seen in the same M-mode view as the mitral valve. In most cases of Ebstein's anomaly the tricuspid valve closes

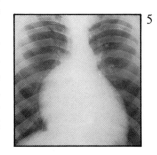

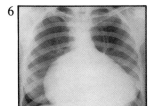

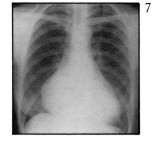

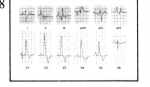

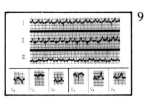

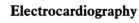

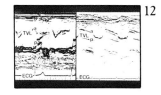

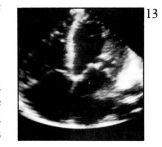

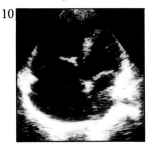

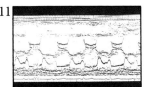

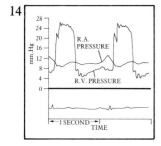

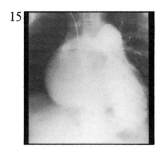

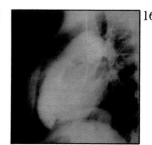

significantly later than the mitral valve [11]. In rheumatic tricuspid valve disease similar abnormalities are seen in the mobility and structure of the tricuspid valve as are seen in rheumatic mitral valve disease [12,13]. The large right atrium may be visualized directly and in pure tricuspid regurgitation the large right ventricle will be seen.

Contrast echocardiography may be useful in the diagnosis of both Ebstein's anomaly and tricuspid regurgitation. The bubbles may be seen to pass from right to left across the atrial septum in Ebstein's anomaly, while in tricuspid regurgitation the bubbles may pass back and forth across the tricuspid valve.

Cardiac Catheterization and Angiography

In Ebstein's anomaly it may be evident at cardiac catheterization that a right atrial pressure trace is obtained in a position when an endocardial electrode shows right ventricular configuration. Tricuspid regurgitation will result in an elevation of mean right atrial pressure with a dominant 'v' wave; the presence of tricuspid stenosis will be detected by simultaneous pressure tracings in the right atrium and right ventricle showing a diastolic pressure difference [14].

Angiography in Ebstein's anomaly will show displacement of the effective right atrioventricular orifice into the cavity of the right ventricle, frequently with atrialization of the ventricular inlet portion. This results in tricuspid regurgitation and a very large right atrium and atrialized portion [15,16].

1   Heart with Ebstein's anomaly of the tricuspid valve viewed from the outlet portion of the right ventricle. The valve is a fenestrated curtain which is attached in such a way as to separate the inlet and outlet portions of the right ventricle. The cavity of the inlet portion (atrialized right ventricle) is behind the valve.

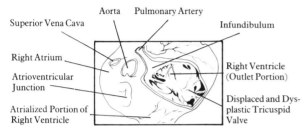

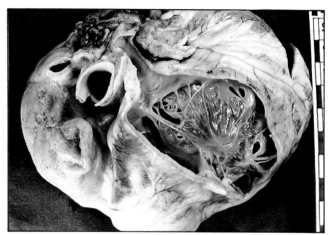

2   Heart viewed from the right atrium with tricuspid stenosis and incompetence due to rheumatic involvement of the valve cusps.

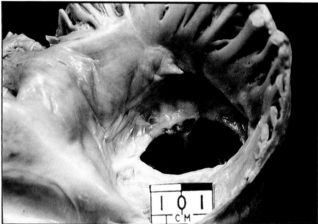

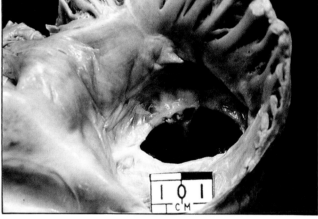

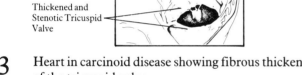

3   Heart in carcinoid disease showing fibrous thickening of the tricuspid valve.

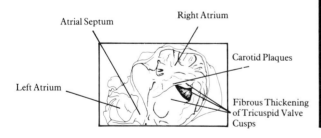

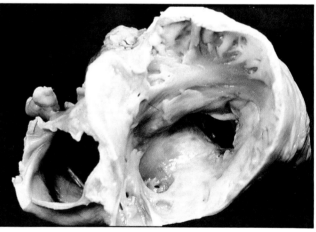

4 Chest radiograph in Ebstein's anomaly. The heart is enlarged and globular. There is a prominent bulge on the left heart border due to the displaced right ventricular outflow tract.

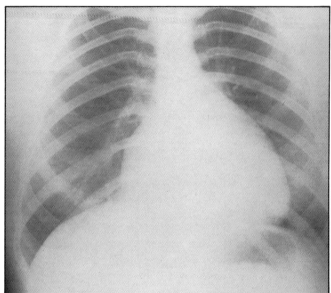

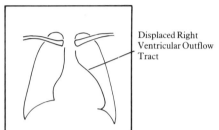

Displaced Right Ventricular Outflow Tract

5 Chest radiograph in Ebstein's anomaly showing pulmonary oligaemia and a prominent right atrial border.

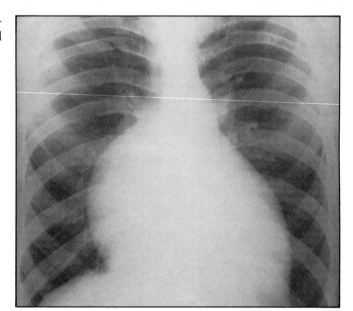

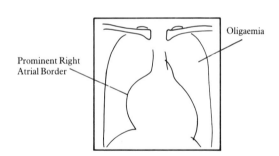

Oligaemia

Prominent Right Atrial Border

6 Chest radiograph in rheumatic tricuspid stenosis showing an enormous right atrium.

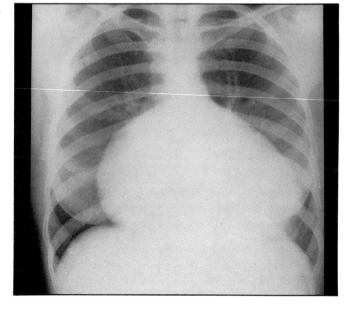

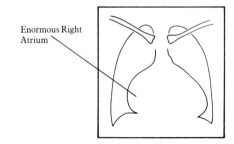

Enormous Right Atrium

TRICUSPID VALVE DISEASE

7   Chest radiograph in rheumatic tricuspid and mitral disease showing a large right atrium. Upper lobe blood diversion is inconspicuous.

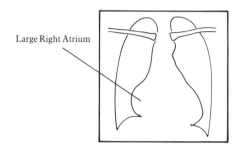

Large Right Atrium

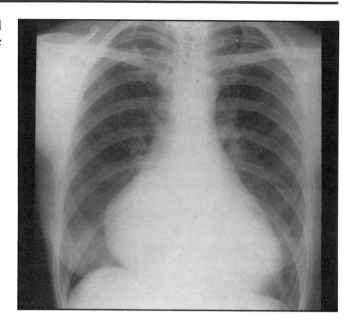

TRICUSPID VALVE DISEASE

8

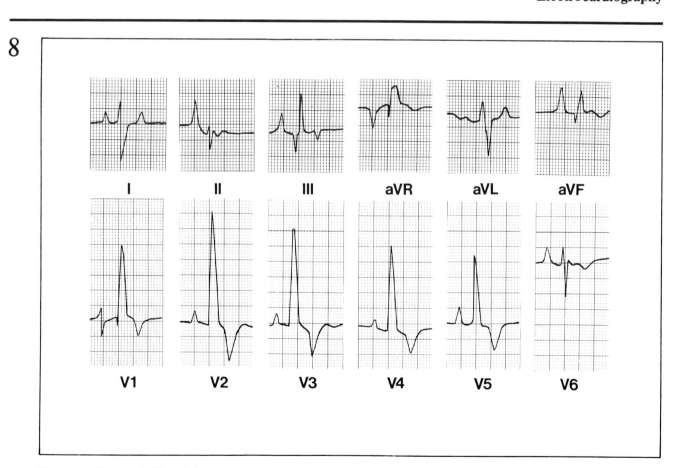

Electrocardiogram in Ebstein's anomaly showing tall P waves and right bundle branch block.

9

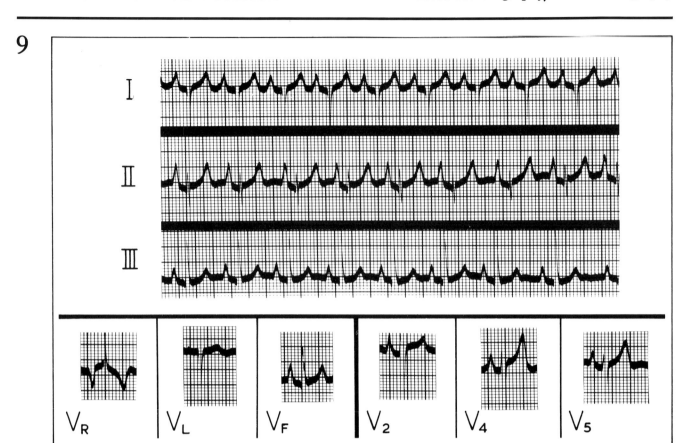

Electrocardiogram in tricuspid stenosis showing right atrial hypertrophy (tall P wave in lead II).

10

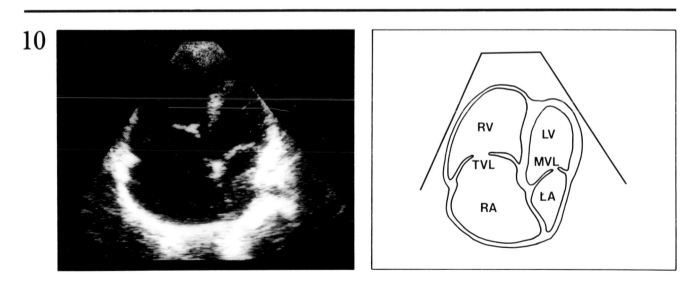

2-D echocardiographic apical four-chamber view of Ebstein's anomaly. The tricuspid valve is greatly displaced into the right ventricle.

11

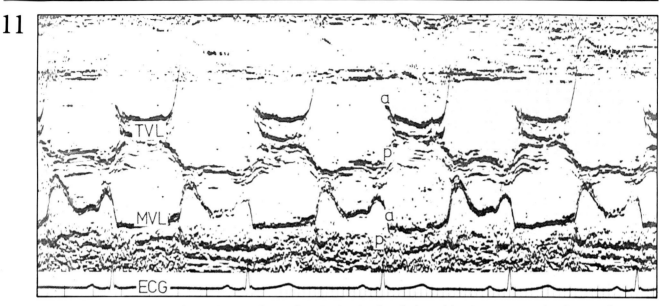

M-mode echocardiogram of Ebstein's malformation. Both mitral and tricuspid valves are seen simultaneously with tricuspid valve closure occurring after mitral valve closure.

12

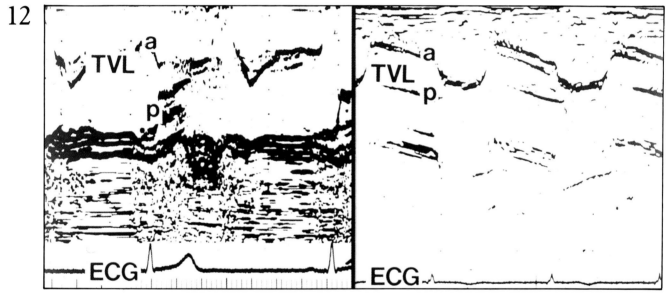

M-mode echocardiogram of tricuspid stenosis (right hand panel) showing reduced diastolic closure rate. A normal tricuspid valve is shown in the left hand panel for comparison.

13

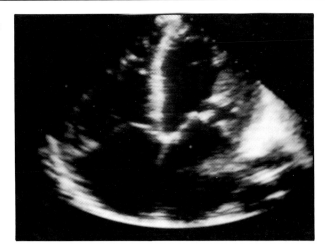
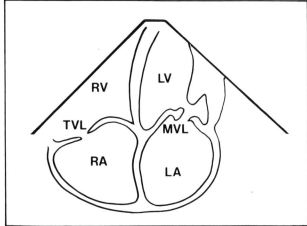

Apical four-chamber 2-D echocardiographic view in rheumatic mitral and tricuspid valve disease. The leaflet tips hardly separate.

TRICUSPID VALVE DISEASE

Cardiac Catheterization & Angiography

14 Pressure tracings from a patient with tricuspid stenosis showing a diastolic gradient between right atrium and right ventricle.

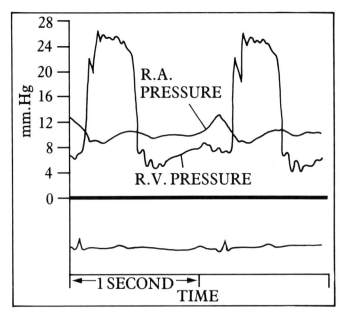

15 Right ventricular angiogram (antero-posterior projection) in Ebstein's anomaly. The injection is in the outlet portion. Both the true atrioventricular annulus and the effective orifice are outlined by regurgitation through the downwardly displaced tricuspid valve. The right atrium is dilated. In this patient there was additional pulmonary valve stenosis.

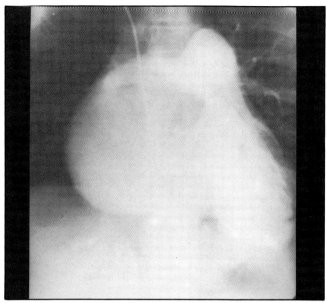

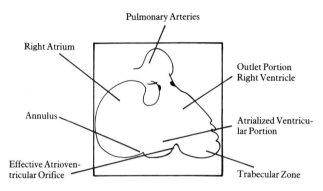

16 Lateral projection of [14]. The effective orifice of the tricuspid valve is seen between the inlet and outlet portions of the right ventricle. The thickened pulmonary valve is also seen.

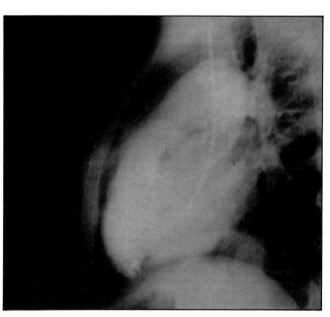

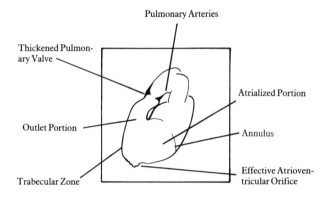

Chapter 5.

Congenital Heart Disease

Abbreviations

Ao	Aorta	LCCA	Left Common Carotid Artery	PVW	Posterior Ventricular Wall
Asc Ao	Ascending Aorta	LPA	Left Pulmonary Artery	RA	Right Atrium
ASD	Atrial Septal Defect	LSA	Left Subclavian Artery	RAVL	Right Atrioventricular Valve Leaflet
AV	Aortic Valve	LV	Left Ventricle		
CW	Chest Wall	MV	Mitral Valve	RPA	Right Pulmonary Artery
Desc Ao	Descending Aorta	MVL	Mitral Valve Leaflet	RV	Right Ventricle
En	Endocardium	PA	Pulmonary Artery	RVOT	Right Ventricular Outflow Tract
Ep	Epicardium	PDA	Persistent Ductus Arteriosus		
Inn	Innominate Artery			S	Septum
IS	Infundibular Stenosis	PT	Pulmonary Trunk	TV	Tricuspid Valve
IVS	Interventricular Septum	PV	Pulmonary Valve	VSD	Ventricular Septal Defect
LA	Left Atrium	PVL	Pulmonary Valve Leaflet		
LAVL	Left Atrioventricular Valve Leaflet				

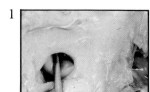

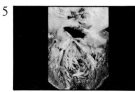

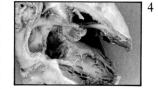

Pathology

In up to 25% of all normal hearts there is a patent foramen ovale [1]. However a shunt from left atrium to right atrium is prevented by a flap valve and a right to left shunt will only occur if the right atrial pressure is raised. A secundum atrial septal defect results from a deficiency of the flap valve of the foramen ovale [2]. Other types of atrial septal defect include 'sinus venosus' defect which lies superior to the fossa ovalis; this is usually associated with partial anomalous pulmonary venous return either into the superior vena cava or into the right atrium [3]. Rarely a defect in the postero-inferior portion of the atrium results in the inferior vena cava draining directly into the left atrium. The ostium primum atrial septal defect usually presenting in childhood involves the lowermost part of the atrial septum [4] and is characteristically associated with a defect of the ventricular septum and cleft in the atrioventricular valves [5].

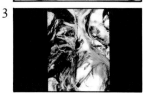

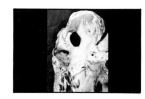

Presentation

Symptoms

Whereas most children with an atrial septal defect are asymptomatic, patients presenting over the age of 40 will often complain of breathlessness on exertion, palpitation or fatigue. Rarely the elderly patient presents not only in atrial fibrillation but with frank heart failure. At any age the lesion may be initially discovered by routine chest x-ray.

Signs

The diagnostic hallmark of an atrial septal defect is the fixed wide splitting of the second heart sound virtually always associated with an ejection systolic murmur in the pulmonary area. Irrespective of the level of the pulmonary artery pressure or the direction of the shunt, pulmonary valve closure is as loud or louder than aortic valve closure. With a large left to right shunt at atrial level there may be an additional mid-diastolic murmur increased by inspiration at the left sternal edge. This is due to increased flow through the normal tricuspid valve. A pan-systolic murmur due to mitral valve regurgitation may suggest ostium primum defect although the electrocardiogram showing left axis deviation will be more helpful. A mid-systolic click and a late systolic murmur suggest mitral valve prolapse; this sometimes occurs with a secundum atrial septal defect.

In an atrial septal defect with the Eisenmenger complex, central cyanosis may be present. The auscultatory signs are similar to those of a secundum atrial septal defect with a large left to right shunt except that a pulmonary ejection sound is frequently heard, pulmonary valve closure is very loud and a tricuspid flow murmur is not present.

The quality of the arterial pulse in an atrial septal defect is usually normal but the jugular venous pulse is frequently visible with a normal wave form unless there is additional tricuspid

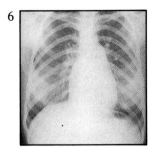

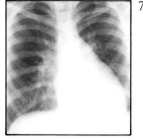

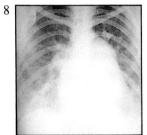

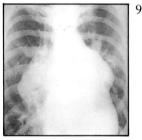

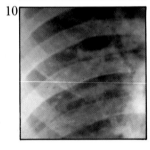

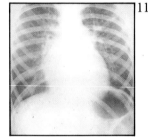

regurgitation. There may be a hyperdynamic impulse at the left sternal edge due to increased right ventricular stroke volume but this finding is often obscured in the elderly patient.

Investigations

Radiology

Both the central and peripheral pulmonary vessels in a left to right shunting atrial septal defect are dilated due to increased pulmonary blood flow (pulmonary plethora) [6]. The aortic knuckle is usually small. Most adults also show cardiac enlargement as a result of right ventricular and right atrial dilatation [7]. If there is marked pulmonary hypertension with a left to right shunt all these features become more obvious [8]. If the Eisenmenger reaction has occurred the central pulmonary arteries may become very large while the distal vessels are reduced in calibre [9]. There may be calcified atheroma in the pulmonary artery. The presence of partial anomalous pulmonary venous drainage may be indicated by the anomalous veins lying in an abnormal anatomical position [10]. Although the chest radiograph of an ostium primum atrial septal defect may be indistinguishable from that of a secundum defect, upper zone vessel dilatation and left atrial enlargment may be apparent, reflecting mitral regurgitation [11].

Electrocardiography

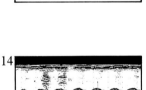

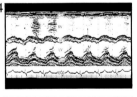

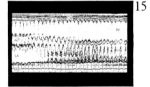

The typical ECG of a secundum atrial septal defect shows a normal QRS axis with complete or incomplete right bundle branch block [12]. There may be frank right ventricular hypertrophy recognized from the ECG in an atrial septal defect with severe pulmonary hypertension. Left axis deviation in the ECG suggests that the atrial septal defect is of the ostium primum variety [13].

Echocardiography

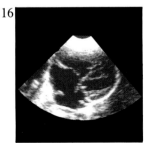

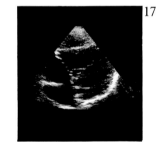

M-mode echocardiography in atrial septal defect shows a dilated right ventricle relative to the left due to the volume overload [14]. This usually results in reversed septal motion [15]. Two-dimensional echocardiography can directly visualize the defects in the majority of cases. The atrial septum is best viewed from the subcostal position and when a secundum defect is present it is seen to lie centrally bounded superiorly and inferiorly by atrial septal tissue and the atrioventricular septum is always intact with a clear separation of the septal insertion of the mitral and tricuspid valves [16]. In an ostium primum defect both mitral and tricuspid valves insert onto the crest of the ventricular septum at the same level without any atrioventricular septum. The abnormal position of the mitral valve in the left ventricular outflow tract can be seen [17]. Sinus venosus defects are difficult to detect and careful exploration of the atrial septum is necessary. The anomalous drainage of the right upper pulmonary vein to the right side of the atrial septum is best appreciated from the suprasternal position.

Echocardiography using a contrast injection may be helpful in the diagnosis of atrial septal defect. A right to left shunt at atrial level will be readily detected by the passage of microbubbles from the right to the left atrium [18].

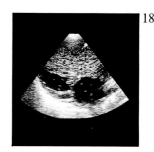

Cardiac Catheterization and Angiography

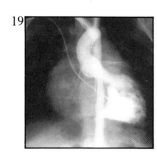

If cardiac catheterization is carried out in patients with atrial septal defects the size of the shunt and its direction will be identified. The level of the pulmonary artery pressure and pulmonary vascular resistance can be measured.

Additional anomalous pulmonary venous drainage can be demonstrated by pulmonary arteriography. In an ostium primum atrial septal defect, left ventricular angiography shows a characteristic abnormality in the left ventricular outflow tract. This is the 'goose-neck' deformity due to the abnormal position of the mitral valve [19].

1 The probe is passed between the flap valve and the limbus. When the probe is removed the flap valve will close the defect.

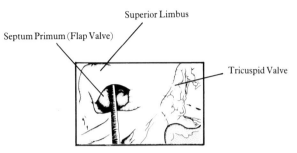

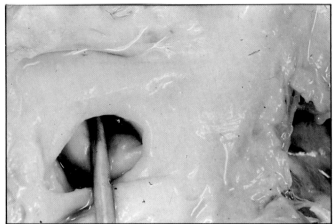

2 Secundum atrial septal defect. A single round defect occupies the site of the foramen ovale. The coronary sinus lies below and the tricuspid valve is separated from the defect by several centimetres of muscle tissue.

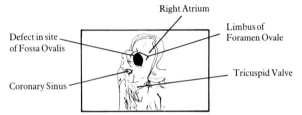

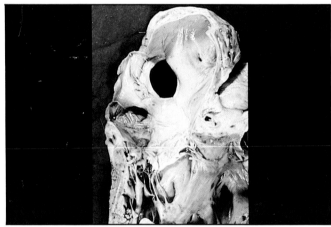

3 Sinus venosus defect. The defect is high in the wall of the superior vena cava and the right pulmonary veins drain to the right atrium via the defect.

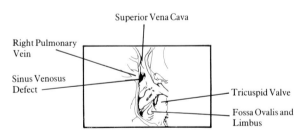

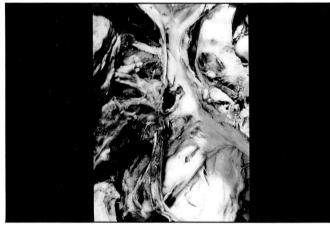

4 The right atrium and ventricle in a heart with an ostium primum atrial septal defect. There is a deficiency in the base of the atrial septum, but separate annuli of the mitral and tricuspid valves.

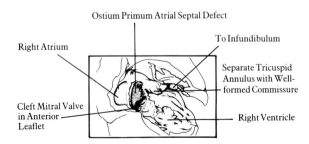

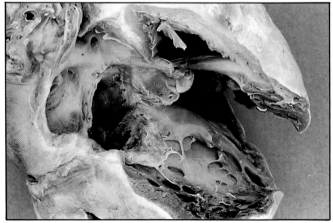

5   The left atrium and ventricle in a heart following operation, with an ostium primum atrial septal defect. There is a cleft in the mitral valve.

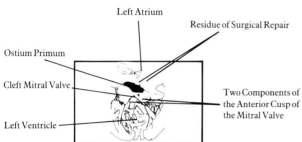

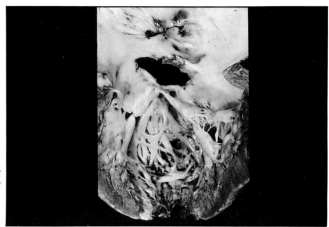

ATRIAL SEPTAL DEFECT

Radiology

6   Chest radiograph in secundum atrial septal defect. There is pulmonary plethora, a large pulmonary trunk and a small aortic knuckle.

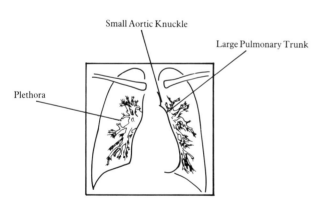

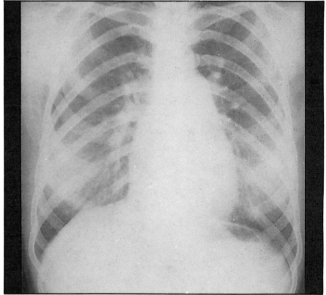

7   Chest radiograph in a secundum atrial septal defect
    showing cardiac enlargement.

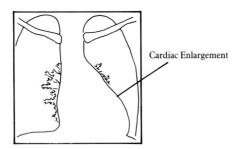

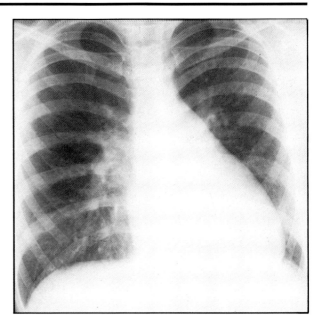

8   Chest radiograph in an atrial septal defect with pul-
    monary hypertension showing a large heart, a grossly
    dilated pulmonary trunk and more obvious plethora.

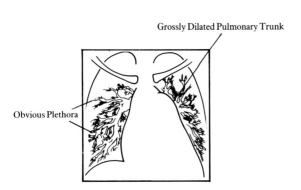

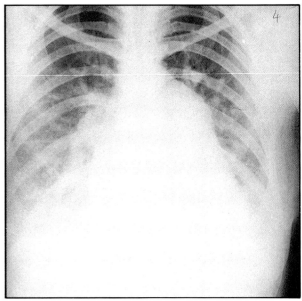

9   Chest radiograph in an atrial septal defect
    complicated by the Eisenmenger reaction. There is
    a grossly dilated pulmonary trunk.

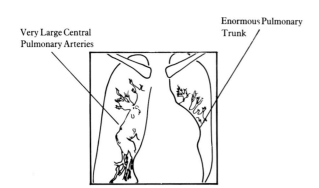

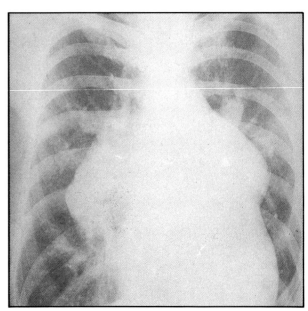

10 Chest radiograph showing a horizontal vessel above the right hilum representing an anomalous pulmonary vein.

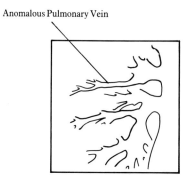

Anomalous Pulmonary Vein

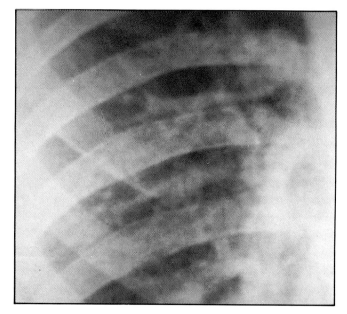

11 Chest radiograph of a primum atrial septal defect with mitral regurgitation showing slight enlargement of the heart, a prominent pulmonary trunk, pulmonary plethora and upper zone vessel dilatation.

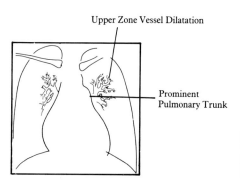

Upper Zone Vessel Dilatation

Prominent Pulmonary Trunk

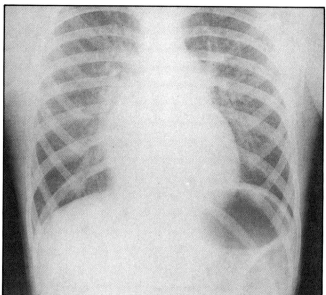

12

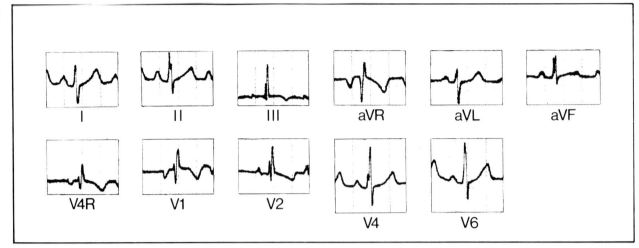

Electrocardiogram of a patient with a secundum atrial septal defect showing sinus rhythm, right axis deviation, and rsR complexes from V4R to V4 indicating incomplete right bundle branch block.

13

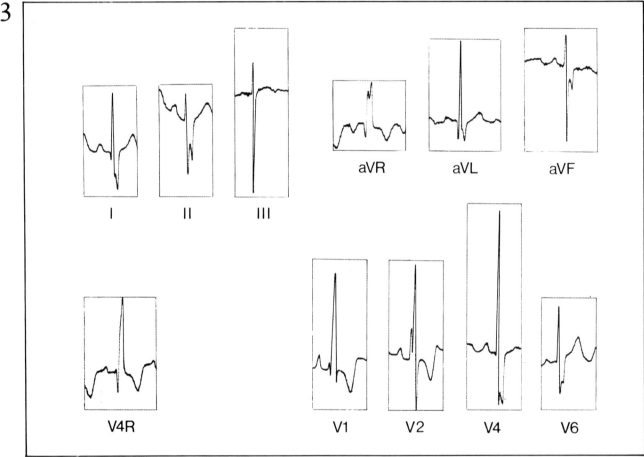

Electrocardiogram of a patient with ostium primum atrial septal defect showing left axis deviation and right bundle branch block.

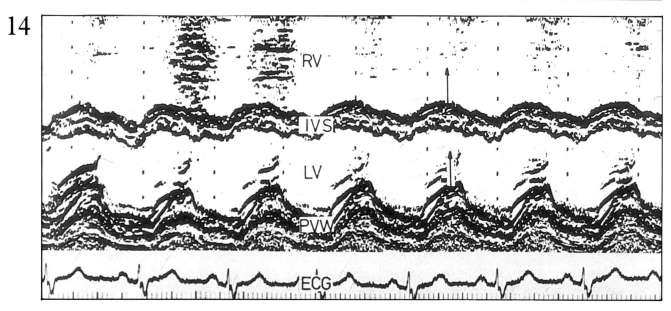

Slow M-mode scan in an atrial septal defect showing the right ventricular enlargement.

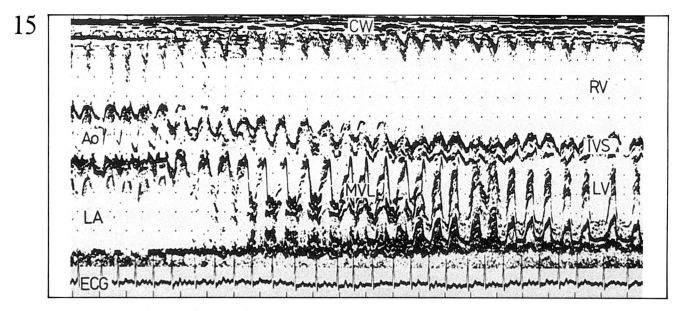

M-mode echocardiogram of a heart with atrial septal defect showing increased right ventricular internal dimension. Left ventricular dimension is smaller than right. Paradoxical septal motion is seen.

16

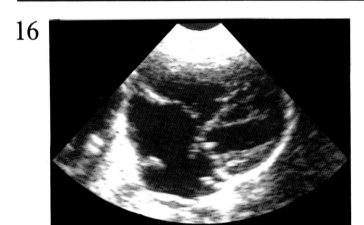 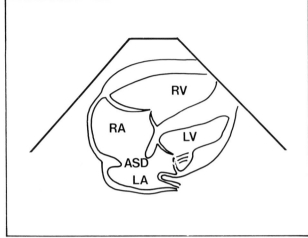

2-D echocardiographic subcostal view showing a secundum atrial septal defect. The defect lies in the central region of the atrial septum and is separated both from the atrioventricular valves and the atrial roof by septal tissue.

17

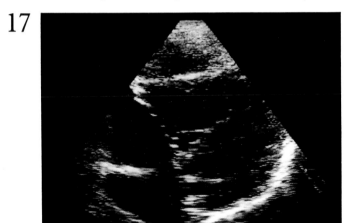 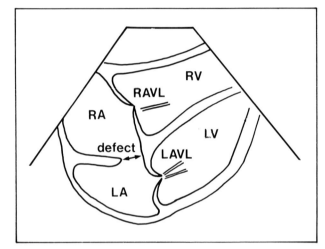

2-D echocardiographic subcostal four-chamber view of an ostium primum atrial septal defect. The defect extends right down to the atrioventricular valve.

18

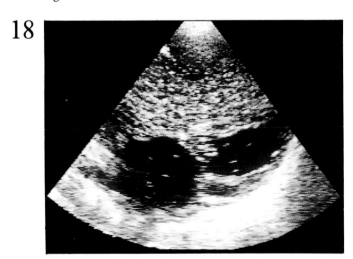 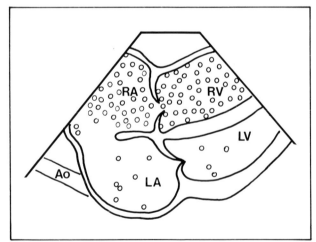

2-D echocardiographic subcostal four-chamber view using a contrast injection. The microbubbles injected into a systemic vein fill the right atrium and right ventricle. Blood shunting left to right shows as an un-opacified region in the right atrium. A few microbubbles are transferred into the left heart indicating that there is also a small right to left shunt.

19 Left ventricular angiogram (antero-posterior projection) in an ostium primum atrial septal defect showing the 'goose-neck' deformity.

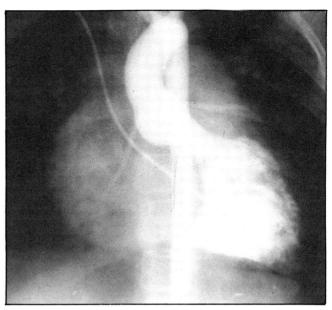

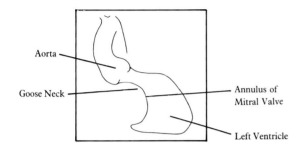

The incidence of ventricular septal defects is 2/1000 live births and constitutes about 20–30% of all congenital cardiac malformations. Its prevalence in school age children is about 1/1000 and in adults approximately 0.5/1000. In the adult it may be a part of a complex congenital cardiac malformation such as Fallot's tetralogy but in this section it will be considered as an isolated abnormality.

Pathology

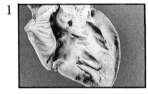
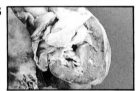
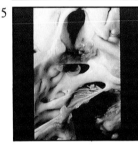
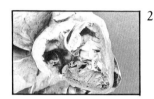
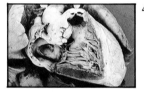
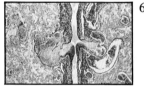

Ventricular septal defects can occur in the membranous septum [1] or in any part of the muscular septum. The defects may be single [2] or multiple [3]. Usually the defect permits communication between the two ventricles, but rarely when the defect is in the atrioventricular component of the membranous septum there will be a communication between the left ventricle and right atrium (Gerbode defect). The most common defects exist in and around the ventricular component of the membranous septum [4]. The size of the defect is variable and the haemodynamic consequences will therefore vary. Defects in the membranous septum are particularly likely to lead to aortic regurgitation due to aortic cusp prolapse [5]. Many of the ventricular septal defects which are present at birth close spontaneously. Later in life, if there has been longstanding left-to-right shunting, pulmonary vascular disease may develop [6].

Infective endocarditis is an important complication even if the lesion is haemodynamically insignificant.

Presentation

Symptoms

The patient with a small left-to-right shunting ventricular septal defect and a normal pulmonary artery pressure (Maladie de Roger) is usually asymptomatic, the condition being diagnosed on routine clinical examination. The child or young adult with a large left-to-right shunt and elevation of the pulmonary artery pressure may complain of breathlessness and fatigue. If pulmonary vascular disease has developed (Eisenmenger ventricular septal defect) then patients may be asymptomatic or complain of breathlessness, fatigue or may even be noticed to be cyanosed.

Signs

The patient with a 'Roger' ventricular septal defect has only a pan-systolic murmur usually accompanied by a thrill at the left sternal edge. The second heart sound may be abnormally widely split in expiration but moves normally in inspiration.

The patient with a large left-to-right shunt and pulmonary hypertension will have a hyperdynamic apical impulse reflecting the increased stroke volume of the left ventricle. On auscultation, in addition to the pan-systolic murmur, the pulmonary valve closure sound is accentuated although the splitting is physiological. There is often an additional mid-diastolic murmur reflecting the increased flow through the normal mitral valve.

The patient with the Eisenmenger ventricular septal defect

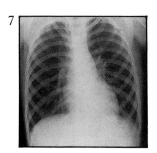

may be cyanosed and clubbed. The jugular venous pulse may show abnormal dominance of the 'a' wave while the arterial pulse is usually normal. On auscultation the characteristic finding is that the second heart sound is single although incorporating both components (aortic closure and pulmonary closure) which have become fused. The second heart sound is accentuated due to the loud pulmonary closure sound. There may be no murmurs but a pulmonary ejection sound and a short ejection systolic murmur are common.

Investigations

Radiology

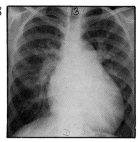

A small ventricular defect does not cause cardiac enlargement, but the central pulmonary arteries are usually slightly enlarged in the plain chest radiograph [7]. With a larger defect there is cardiac enlargement. The increased pulmonary flow and pressure is reflected in left atrial dilatation, a large pulmonary trunk and obvious pulmonary plethora [8]. If pulmonary vascular disease has developed (Eisenmenger situation) there is enlargement of the pulmonary trunk and central pulmonary vessels [9], while the peripheral vessels are constricted.

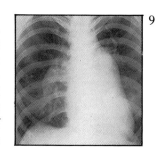

Electrocardiography

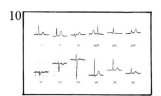

In a small left-to-right shunting defect the electrocardiogram may be normal. The adult with a moderately large left-to-right shunting defect may show voltage increases (tall R-waves in V5 and S-waves in V1) indicating left ventricular enlargement [10]. The electrocardiogram in a defect complicated by the Eisenmenger reaction shows right ventricular hypertrophy [11] although additional left ventricular hypertrophy is often also seen.

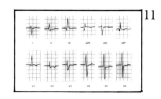

Echocardiography

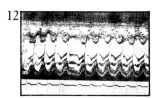

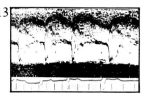

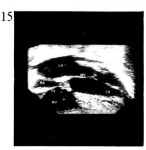

Although M-mode echocardiography provides information about the dimensions of the ventricles it does not enable the ventricular septal defect to be visualized directly. Thus in small defects the M-mode echocardiogram is frequently normal. With larger shunts the M-mode features are those of left ventricular volume overload (increased left ventricular end-diastolic and left atrial dimensions) [12]. In the presence of the Eisenmenger situation the right ventricular dimension is also increased and the pulmonary valve echocardiogram is abnormal. Abnormalities of the pulmonary valve which suggest pulmonary hypertension include flattening of the diastolic line, absence of the 'a' dip, large amplitude of systolic opening and mid-systolic vibration and partial collapse [13]. While none of these features taken in isolation are diagnostic, the presence of all strongly suggest significant pulmonary hypertension.

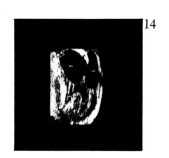

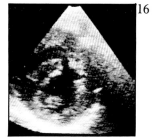

Two-dimensional echocardiography has proved extremely valuable in the identification of ventricular septal defects. Careful use of various views show characteristic features in many of the different anatomical locations of the defects. Thus a subcostal four-chamber view enables a perimembranous [14] or inlet muscular [15] ventricular septal defect to be visualized. A parasternal short axis view may enable an anterior trabecular muscular defect to be seen [16].

Cardiac Catheterization and Angiography

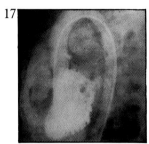

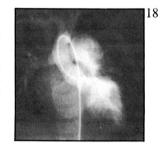

The left-to-right shunt or bi-directional shunt can be detected at cardiac catheterization and the pulmonary artery pressure measured. Pulmonary vascular resistance and pulmonary to systemic flow ratios may be calculated. A left ventricular angiogram shows the position of the ventricular septal defect and whether multiple defects are present [17,18,19].

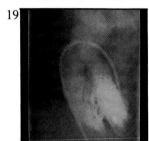

1 Heart from which the parietal wall of the right ventricle has been removed showing a slit-like defect at the site of the membranous septum.

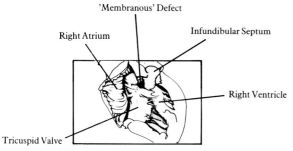

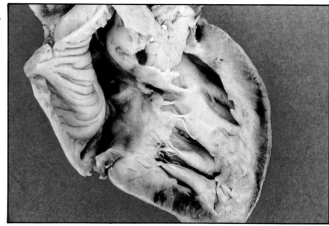

2 Posterior muscular septal defect.

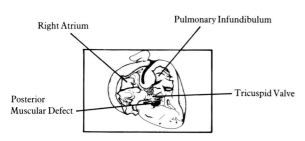

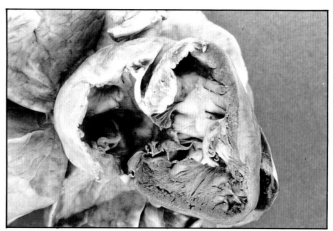

3 Multiple muscular defects in trabecular septum.

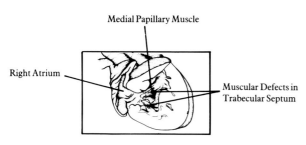

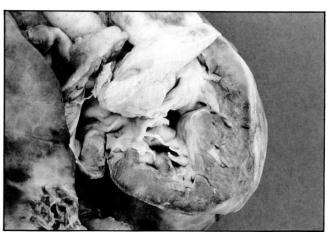

4 Heart opened in a similar fashion to [1] showing a large defect of the muscle surrounding the membranous septum.

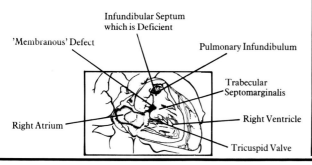

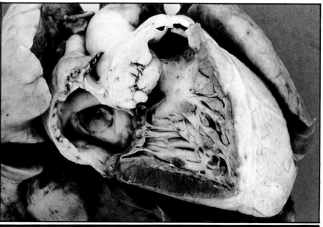

5 Infundibular septal defect with prolapsing aortic valve leaflet.

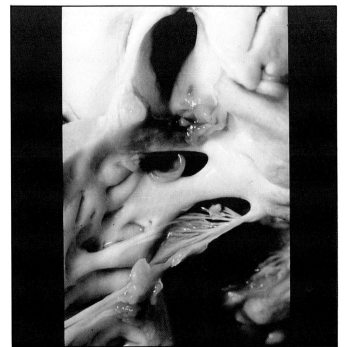

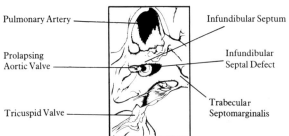

Pulmonary Artery

Prolapsing Aortic Valve

Tricuspid Valve

Infundibular Septum

Infundibular Septal Defect

Trabecular Septomarginalis

6 Pulmonary vascular disease secondary to a ventricular septal defect.

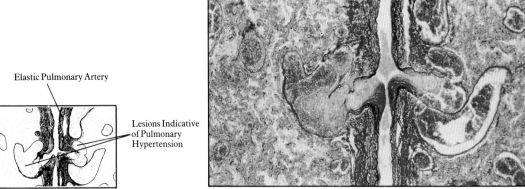

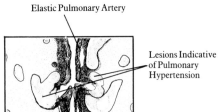

Elastic Pulmonary Artery

Lesions Indicative of Pulmonary Hypertension

7 Chest radiograph showing normal sized heart with slight enlargement of the central pulmonary arteries in a small ventricular septal defect.

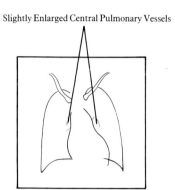

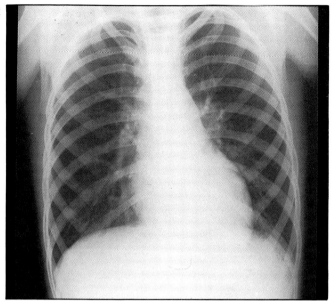

8 Chest radiograph showing increased cardiac size with dilatation of the left atrium, pulmonary trunk and pulmonary plethora in a ventricular septal defect with pulmonary hypertension.

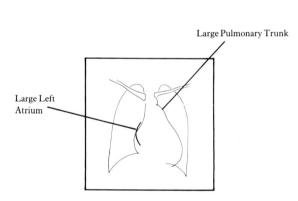

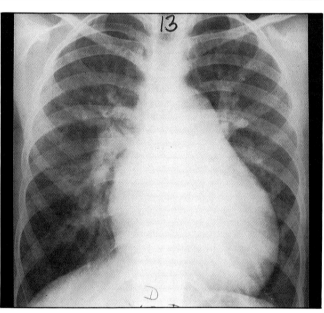

9 Chest radiograph in Eisenmenger ventricular septal defect showing slight enlargement of the heart and gross enlargement of the central pulmonary vessels.

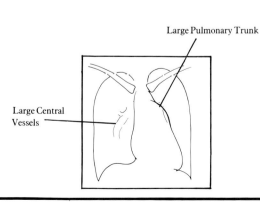

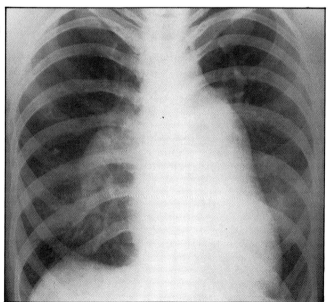

10

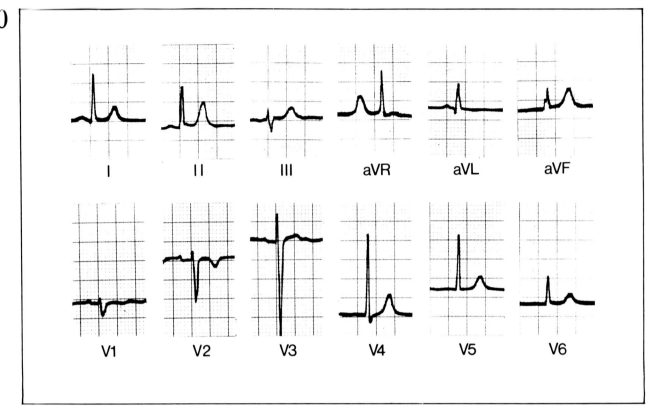

Electrocardiogram of a 10-year-old patient with ventricular septal defect. The pulmonary systemic flow ratio was 2:1 and the pulmonary vascular resistance normal. There is evidence of slight left ventricular hypertrophy as shown by the increased voltage of R-waves in the left precordial leads. Note: V4 to V6, 1mV = 0.5 cm.

11

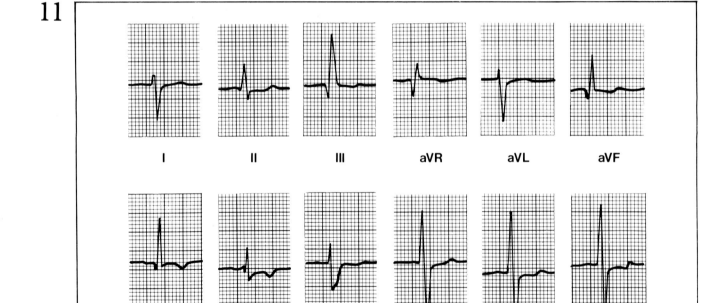

Electrocardiogram of a patient aged 21 with Eisenmenger ventricular septal defect, showing right axis deviation, with dominant R-waves, inverted T-waves in right chest leads and deep S-waves in V5 and V6. Note: 1mV = 0.5 cm.

12

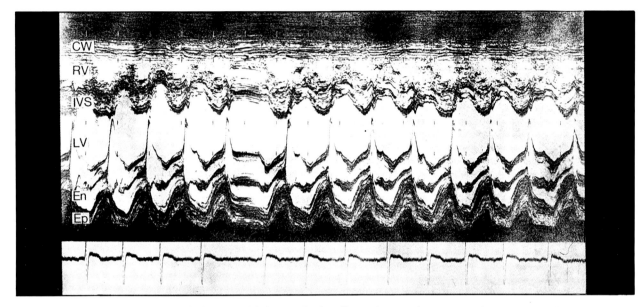

M-mode echocardiogram showing increased left ventricular dimensions and exaggerated movement of the septum and posterior wall in a case of ventricular septal defect with a large shunt.

13

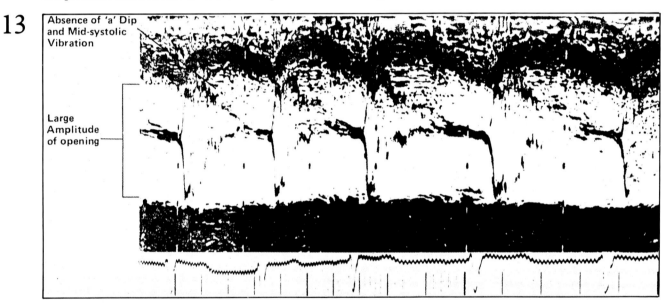

M-mode echocardiogram in ventricular septal defect with severe pulmonary hypertension showing the pulmonary valve. Note the absence of the 'a' dip, large amplitude of systolic opening and partial collapse and vibration of the pulmonary valve in mid-systole.

14

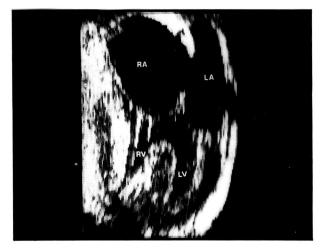 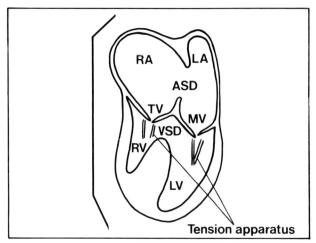

2-D echocardiographic subcostal four-chamber section close to the crux of the heart showing a perimembranous defect situated between the ventricular inlet components. The defect is roofed by the tricuspid and mitral valves in fibrous continuity, the hallmark of this type of defect. There is also an atrial septal defect within the fossa ovalis. Note that the tension apparatus is also seen.

15

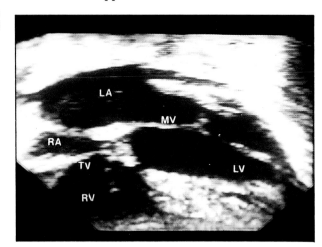 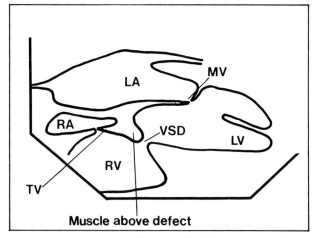

2-D echocardiographic subcostal four-chamber section showing a muscular inlet defect. It is distinguished from the perimembranous defect shown in [14] because it is surrounded by muscle and does not border on the valve annuli. The valve leaflets show the normal off-setting which is lacking in the perimembranous defect.

16

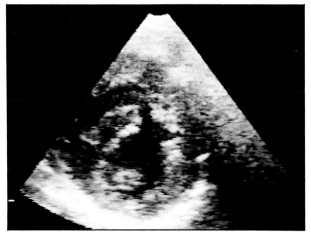 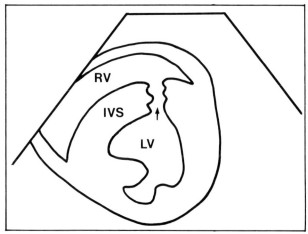

2-D echocardiographic parasternal short axis view showing an anterior trabecular ventricular septal defect (arrowed).

17 Left ventriculogram (lateral projection) showing membranous ventricular septal defect.

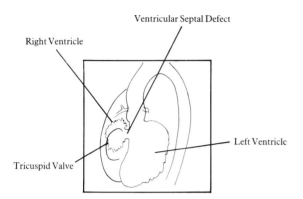

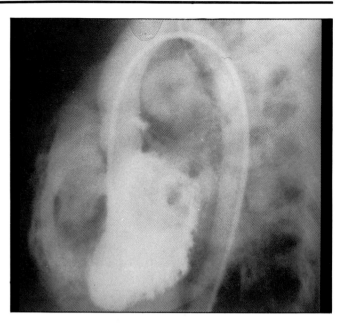

18 Left ventriculogram (antero-posterior projection) showing infundibular septal defect with shunt directly into the pulmonary trunk. The body of the right ventricle is not filled.

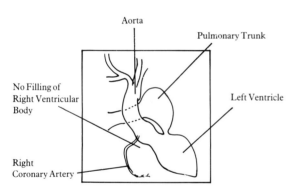

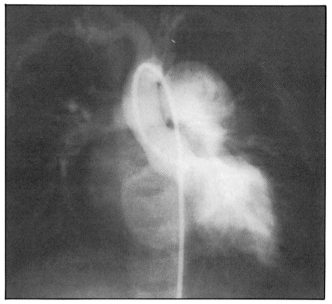

19 Left ventriculogram viewed in a projection which profiles the septum showing multiple defects in the trabecular septum.

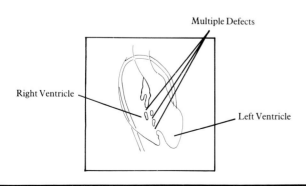

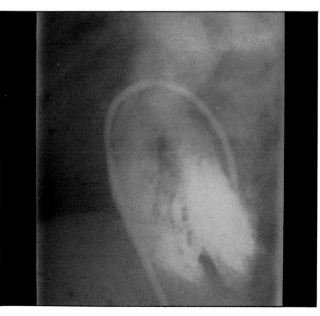

Pathology

The ductus arteriosus connects the proximal left pulmonary artery to the arch of the aorta just distal to the origin of the left subclavian artery and forms a communication between the pulmonary and systemic circulation which persists throughout the whole of foetal life and into the neonatal period [1]. Normally it closes shortly after birth but it may, for reasons which are not fully understood, remain patent throughout life. In children who have a persistent ductus arteriosus a small proportion will have an additional cardiac abnormality.

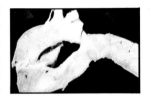

Presentation

Symptoms

The lesion is rare in adults because it has usually been corrected by surgery in childhood. Adults presenting with isolated persistent ductus arteriosus are usually asymptomatic and discovered by the chance finding of a murmur. Patients with a longstanding large left-to-right shunt may complain of breathlessness and even develop frank heart failure particularly following the development of atrial fibrillation.

Signs

The physical signs of a left-to-right shunting persistent ductus arteriosus include a continuous murmur best heard in the left infraclavicular area. If the shunt is small there may be no other abnormal physical signs; if the shunt is large there may be a sharp upstroke to the carotid pulse and a hyperdynamic left ventricle on palpation. Additionally there may be a mid-diastolic flow murmur in the mitral area. If pulmonary hypertension is present, the pulmonary valve closure sound will be accentuated.

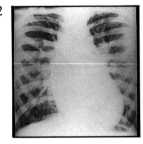

The patient presenting with the Eisenmenger reaction and a persistent ductus arteriosus may be cyanosed particularly in the lower limbs with clubbing of the toes. The remaining physical signs include a physiological splitting of the second heart sound but with an accentuated pulmonary valve closure sound, and right ventricular hypertrophy on palpation. There may be abnormal dominance of the 'a' wave in the jugular venous pulse. There may be either a short ejection systolic murmur or no murmur at all, but a pulmonary ejection sound may be present. An early diastolic murmur due to pulmonary regurgitation may be heard in those patients with the greatest dilatation of the central pulmonary arteries.

Investigations

Radiology

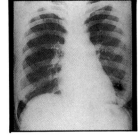

The patient with the large left-to-right shunt may show pulmonary plethora together with cardiac enlargement [2]. Characteristically the aorta is dilated at the site of the ductus [3]. The older patient may show calcification in the region of the ductus [4].

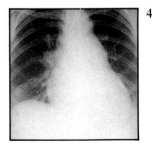

The patient with the Eisenmenger persistent ductus arteriosus

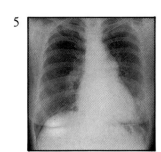

may have a normal sized heart but with dilated central pulmonary arteries and reduction in calibre of the peripheral pulmonary arteries [5].

Electrocardiography

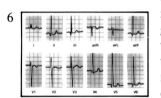

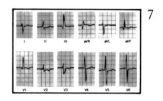

If the ductus is small, the electrocardiogram will be normal. If the shunt is large, the left ventricle dilates and the electrocardiogram may show tall R-waves in V5 and deep S-waves in V1 (voltage changes of left ventricular hypertrophy) [6]. With the development of severe pulmonary vascular disease, the electrocardiogram reflects increasing right ventricular hypertrophy with tall R-waves and T-wave inversion in right ventricular leads and deep S-waves in the left ventricular leads [7]. Right axis deviation and right bundle-branch block are also common features in persistent ductus with severe pulmonary vascular disease.

Echocardiography

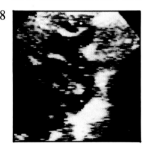

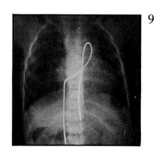

It is possible to identify a persistent ductus arteriosus directly using two-dimensional echocardiography from the suprasternal position [8]. Patients with a large left-to-right shunt will show increase in left ventricular end-diastolic dimension consistent with an increase in stroke volume. The older patient may also show a large left atrium.

Cardiac Catheterization and Angiography

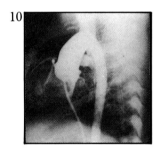

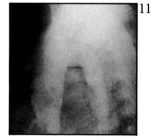

Evidence of a left-to-right shunt can be detected by a step up in oxygen saturation in the pulmonary artery. The catheter can usually be passed directly from the left pulmonary artery into the descending aorta via the ductus arteriosus [9]. The presence of increased pulmonary artery pressure or increased pulmonary vascular resistance can be measured directly.

The aortogram is used to show the anatomy of the ductus [10,11].

PERSISTENT DUCTUS ARTERIOSUS

1   Pathological specimen showing a persistent ductus arteriosus.

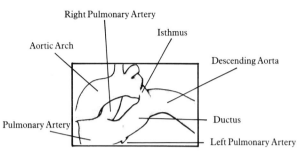

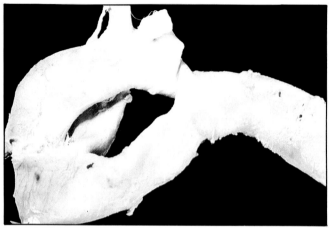

PERSISTENT DUCTUS ARTERIOSUS

2   Chest radiograph in persistent ductus arteriosus with a large left-to-right shunt showing a large heart and pulmonary trunk, prominent aortic knuckle and obvious pulmonary plethora.

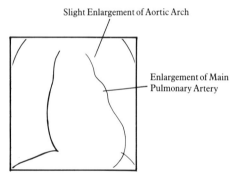

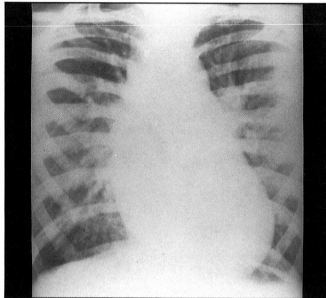

3 Chest radiograph showing a dilated aorta at the site of the persistent ductus.

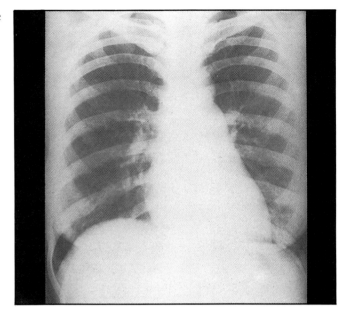

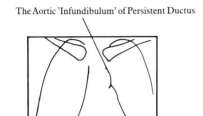

The Aortic 'Infundibulum' of Persistent Ductus

4 Chest radiograph showing calcification in the aorta at the orifice of a persistent ductus.

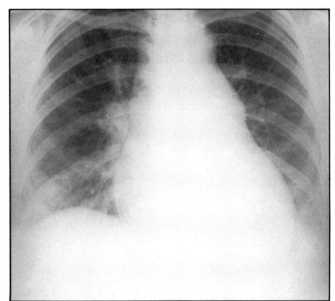

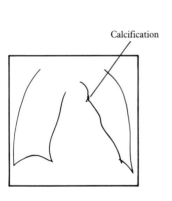

Calcification

5 Chest radiograph in persistent ductus with the Eisenmenger situation showing a slightly enlarged heart, very large pulmonary trunk and prominent aortic knuckle. The hilar vessels are large and the peripheral pulmonary vessels normal.

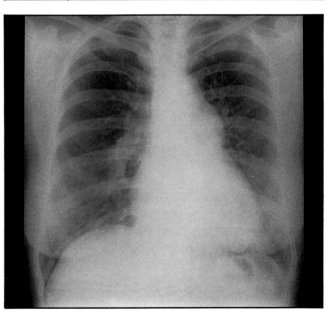

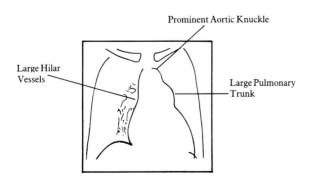

Prominent Aortic Knuckle

Large Hilar Vessels

Large Pulmonary Trunk

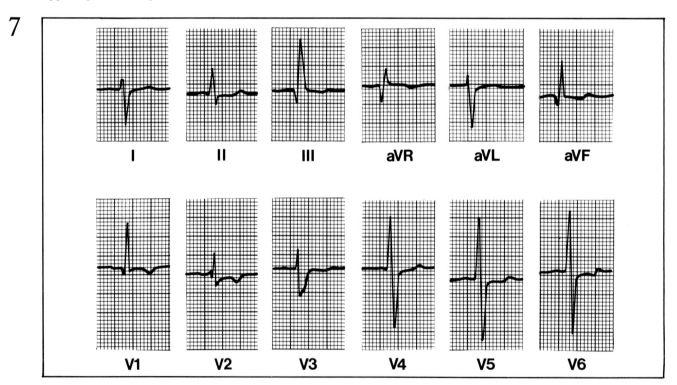

6

Electrocardiogram in persistent ductus arteriosus showing tall R-waves in left ventricular leads and deep S waves in opposing leads - the pattern of diastolic overload.

7

Electrocardiogram in Eisenmenger persistent ductus arteriosus, showing right axis deviation, dominant R-waves, inverted T-waves in right chest leads and deep S-waves in V5 and V6. Note 1 mV = 0.5 cm.

8

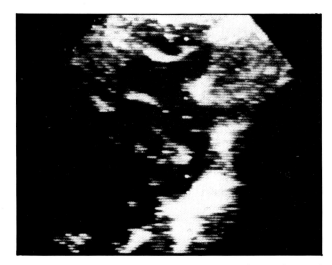
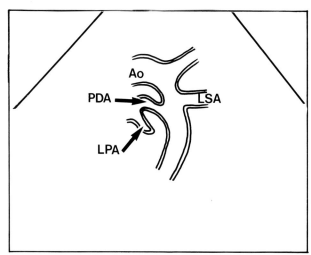

Suprasternal 2-D echocardiographic view of a persistent ductus arteriosus. The duct originates at the level of the left subclavian artery (LSA) and inserts into the main pulmonary artery.

PERSISTENT DUCTUS ARTERIOSUS

Cardiac Catheterization & Angiography

9 Chest radiograph showing typical position of a cardiac catheter passed across a persistent ductus from the pulmonary trunk to the descending aorta.

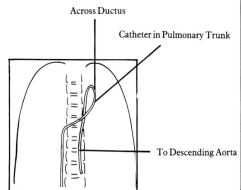
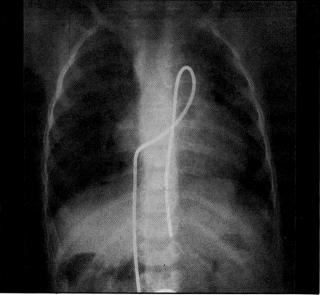

10   Aortogram (lateral projection) showing a small persistent ductus.

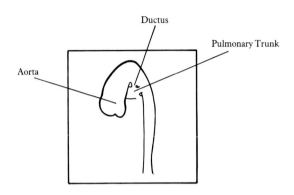

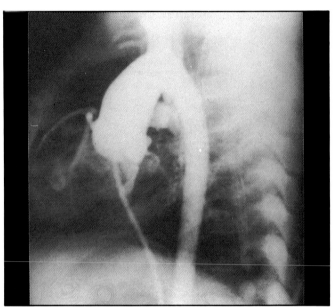

11   Aortogram (lateral projection) showing a large ductus.

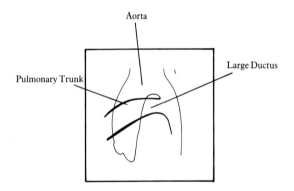

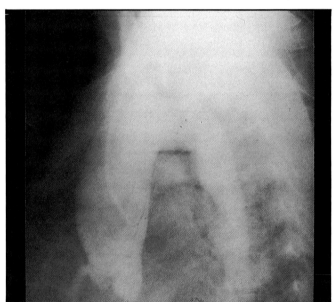

Pathology

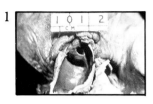

Right ventricular outflow tract obstruction can occur either at pulmonary valve level or due to narrowing of the infundibular portion of the right ventricle or both. In pulmonary valve stenosis the valve is usually tricuspid and the valve cusps are fused along the margins to form an obstructing diaphragm [1]. The valve orifice size may vary from 2–10 mm in diameter [2]. The valve may tend to become thickened and calcified. Right ventricular hypertrophy will develop with time even if the orifice is mildly narrowed [3]. Dilatation of the pulmonary arteries beyond the valve occurs gradually. Rarely, pulmonary valve stenosis may be due to the carcinoid syndrome.

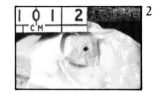

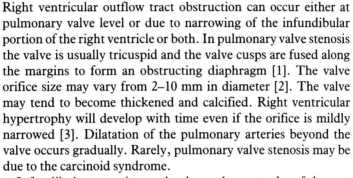

Infundibular stenosis may be due to hypertrophy of the outflow tract [3]. Obstruction may rarely occur if there is a compression externally from a tumour or aberrant muscle bundle within the right ventricle. Infundibular stenosis may develop in patients with a large left to right shunt due to ventricular septal defect, or may be present in hypertrophic cardiomyopathy.

Presentation

Symptoms

The majority of adults with pulmonary valve stenosis, even with significant obstruction, deny symptoms. Occasionally patients may complain of fatigue or dyspnoea. The presence of angina or syncope would indicate severe obstruction as would the development of right heart failure.

Signs

Most patients with right ventricular outflow obstruction presenting in adult life are detected because of the chance finding of a murmur. The murmur is ejection in type and finishes before pulmonary valve closure. In mild or moderate pulmonary valve stenosis, the second heart sound is abnormally widely split in expiration, though the split widens further on inspiration as would occur in normal patients. The severity of the stenosis determines the width of splitting: the wider the expiratory split, the more severe the stenosis. Pulmonary valve closure becomes inaudible when the stenosis is very severe. The abrupt halting of the abnormal pulmonary valve at the onset of systole gives rise to a pulmonary ejection sound. In infundibular stenosis the ejection sound will be absent. Associated right ventricular hypertrophy may be detected by palpation and would give rise to abnormal dominance of the 'a' wave in the venous pulse.

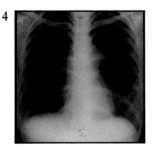

Investigations

Radiology

Pulmonary valve stenosis is characterized on the chest x-ray by a normal sized heart with post-stenotic dilatation of the pulmonary trunk, characteristically extending into the left branch [4]. Pulmonary artery dilatation in some cases may be gross [5]. Pulmonary oligaemia may sometimes be visible.

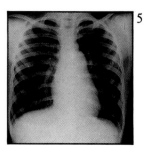

Electrocardiography

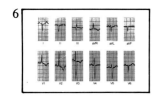

The electrocardiogram in mild or moderate pulmonary stenosis may be normal. In severe pulmonary stenosis, right ventricular hypertrophy is usually present [6]. In severe cases with right heart dilatation, right atrial enlargement may be present in addition to right ventricular hypertrophy.

Echocardiography

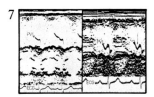

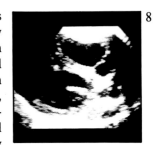

In mild pulmonary valve stenosis, the M-mode echocardiogram is normal. With moderate or severe obstruction the pulmonary valve echo shows marked exaggeration of its 'a' dip [7,8] and in extreme cases the valve may appear to open completely after atrial contraction and before the R wave of the electrocardiogram. In most cases of pulmonary valve stenosis even when it is severe, there is no M-mode echocardiographic evidence of right ventricular hypertrophy but occasionally the septum is thickened and echoes from the anterior wall of the right ventricle are unusually prominent. The septal motion is normal in direction unless the right ventricle fails with secondary tricuspid incompetence. Using two-dimensional echocardiography it may be possible to visualize the thickened restricted domed pulmonary valve. Right ventricular hypertrophy and infundibular obstruction, if present, may also be seen.

Cardiac Catheterization and Angiography

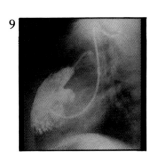

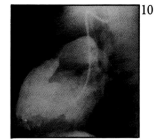

The right ventricular outflow tract obstruction is detected at cardiac catheterization by a systolic pressure difference. The site of obstruction will also be determined.

On right ventricular angiography the site of the outflow obstruction can be seen when it is at valve level [9], infundibular level or in the right ventricular cavity. In pulmonary valve stenosis the cusps will be thickened, domed in systole, with a central jet and post-stenotic dilatation of the pulmonary artery [10].

1 Moderate pulmonary valve stenosis viewed from above, through the opened pulmonary artery.

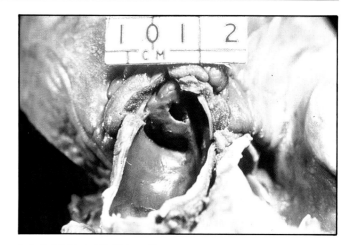

Pulmonary Valve

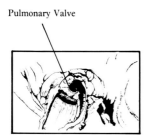

2 Severe pulmonary valve stenosis viewed from above, through the opened pulmonary artery.

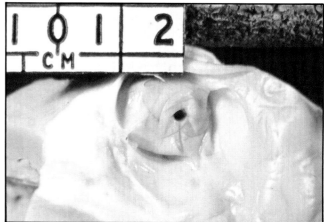

Pulmonary Valve

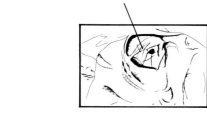

3 Critical pulmonary valve stenosis (red arrow) and secondary infundibular stenosis (white arrow) due to gross right ventricular hypertrophy, the wall being over 1 cm in thickness.

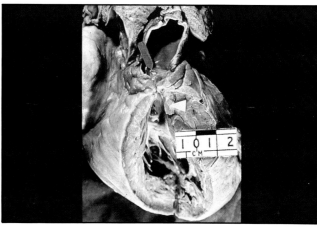

Pulmonary Artery

Critical Pulmonary Valve Stenosis

Secondary Infundibular Stenosis

Hypertrophied Right Ventricle

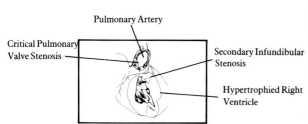

4   Chest radiograph in mild pulmonary stenosis showing post-stenotic dilatation of the pulmonary trunk and a prominent left pulmonary artery.

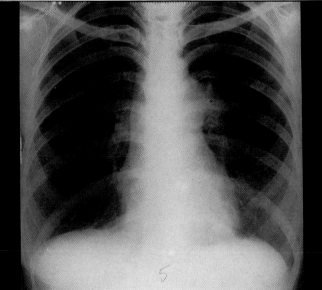

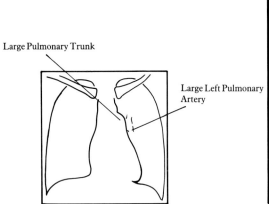

5   Chest radiograph showing obvious post-stenotic dilatation of the left pulmonary artery in pulmonary valve stenosis.

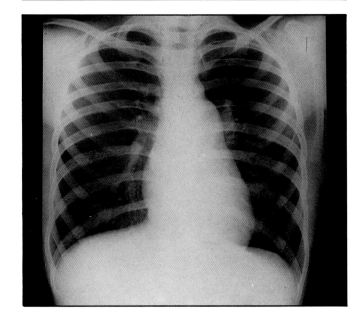

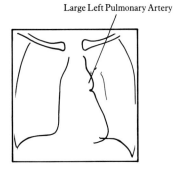

6

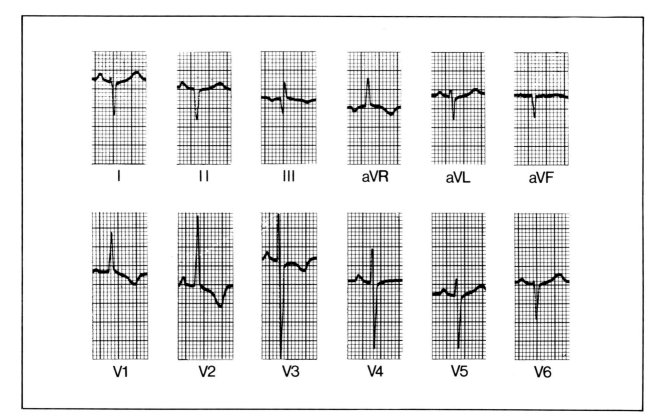

Electrocardiogram in severe pulmonary valve stenosis, showing deep S-wave in lead 1, a dominant R-wave in V1 and T-wave inversion in right chest leads.

7

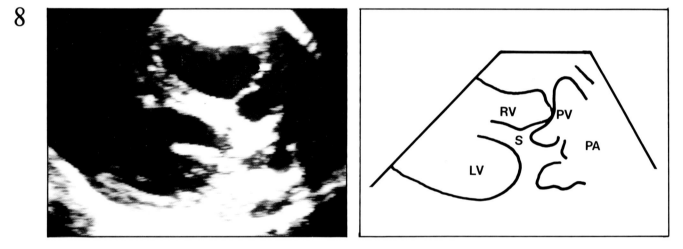

M-mode echocardiogram of the pulmonary valve showing normal atrial dip (Left hand panel; arrowed) and exaggerated atrial dip (arrowed) in pulmonary valve stenosis (right hand panel).

8

2-D echocardiographic view showing thickened pulmonary valve in mild pulmonary stenosis.

9 Right ventricular angiogram (lateral projection) in pulmonary valve stenosis showing a thickened and domed valve with a central systolic jet.

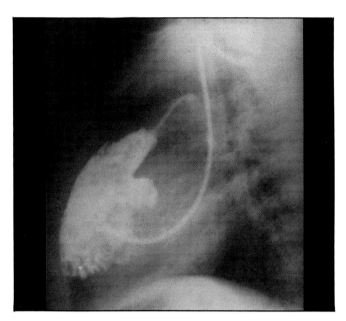

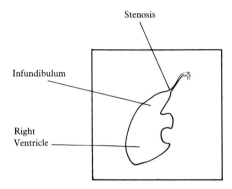

10 Another frame from the same patient as above, showing post-stenotic dilatation of the pulmonary artery.

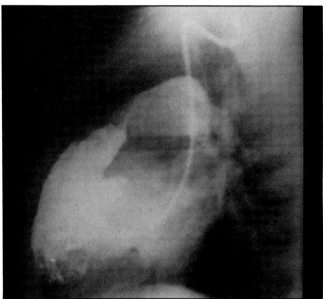

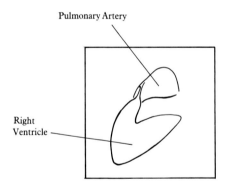

FALLOT'S TETRALOGY

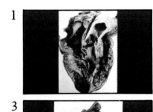

Pathology

Fallot's tetralogy consists of 4 discrete anatomical lesions: pulmonary infundibular stenosis with or without valvular stenosis, a ventricular septal defect, an aorta which overrides the ventricular septum and right ventricular hypertrophy [1,2,3]. The foramen ovale frequently remains patent although contributing little to the main right-to-left shunt which occurs at ventricular level. A right-sided aortic arch persists in 25% of patients.

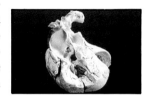

Presentation

Symptoms

Fallot's tetralogy will invariably present and be diagnosed in childhood. In adult life the major complications include cerebral thrombosis (associated with polycythaemia), cerebral abscess, infective endocarditis and rarely cyanotic spells. Paradoxical embolism may occur in Fallot's tetralogy.

Signs

In Fallot's tetralogy the 'a' wave in the venous pulse is not exaggerated because of the associated ventricular septal defect. Usually, there is an ejection systolic murmur which may become abbreviated with severe obstruction. The pulmonary ejection sound and the pulmonary valve closure sound are often not heard as the valve is immobile. Central cyanosis and clubbing are an integral part of the condition.

Investigations

Radiology

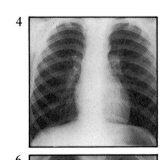

The radiological features of Fallot's tetralogy are a cardiac silhouette of normal size and lung fields which are either normally vascularized or under-vascularized[4]. The cardiac silhouette will not be enlarged in this condition since chamber dilatation is negligible. The shape of the cardiac silhouette is normal in about half the cases and the remainder show a 'boot shape' [5]. This is produced by the hypertrophy of the right ventricle in the absence of left ventricular enlargement leading to a lifting of the apex away from the left dome of the diaphragm, combined with an absence of shadow normally produced by the pulmonary artery (the pulmonary artery in Fallot's tetralogy being small). The absence of shadows in this area may be even more striking when a right-sided aortic arch is present [6].

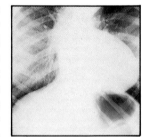

Electrocardiography

In Fallot's tetralogy the electrocardiogram will show moderate right ventricular hypertrophy usually less striking than in severe pulmonary valve stenosis without ventricular septal defect. Right atrial hypertrophy is also less common in Fallot's tetralogy than in pulmonary valve stenosis [7].

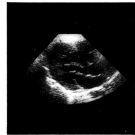

Echocardiography

The characteristic echocardiographic feature of Fallot's tetralogy is overriding of the interventricular septum by the aortic root. This is usually recognizable from the echocardiogram and represents a defect of the infundibular septum. Using 2-dimensional echocardiography both the valvar and infundibular obstruction and the aortic override can be visualized directly as can the ventricular septal defect [8,9].

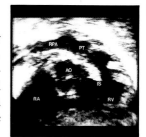

Cardiac Catheterization and Angiography

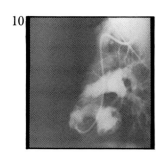

Evidence of a right-to-left shunt at ventricular level will be seen from the desaturation of the left ventricular and aortic blood. A systolic pressure difference will be seen between the right ventricular outlow tract and pulmonary artery.

On right ventricular angiography the outflow tract obstruction can be seen as can the right-to-left shunt across the ventricular septal defect by the passage of contrast from right ventricle to left ventricle [10]. The aortic override infundibular stenosis will also be seen [10,11].

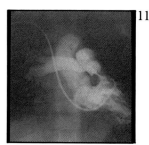

1 Right ventricular view of a specimen with Fallot's tetralogy. The aorta is seen overriding the ventricular septal defect and the infundibular septum is deviated anteriorly to produce infundibular pulmonary stenosis.

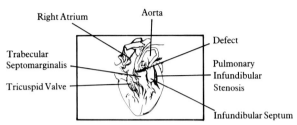

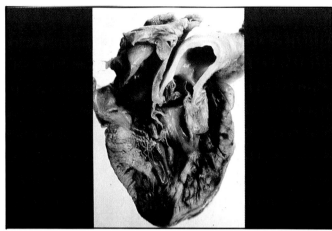

2 Fallot's tetralogy viewed from the anterior aspect with the anterior wall of the right ventricle cut away. Due to extreme aortic override, the great arteries have a side-by-side relationship.

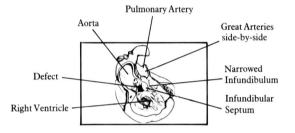

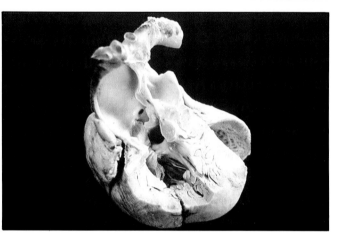

3 Fallot's tetralogy viewed from the right aspect showing extreme anterior deviation of the infundibular septum. The right ventricular outflow tract is a slit (arrowed).

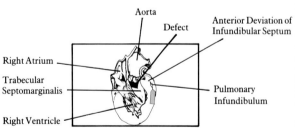

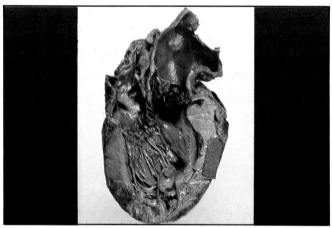

4   Chest radiograph in Fallot's tetralogy showing normal appearance apart from a slightly prominent aorta.

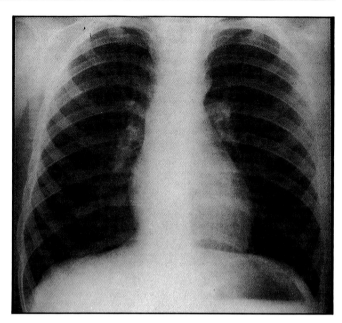

Slightly Prominent Aorta

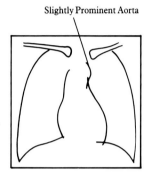

5   Chest radiograph of Fallot's tetralogy showing a typical cardiac silhouette produced by 1) the tipped-up apex, 2) prominent pulmonary bay due to a small pulmonary artery and 3) underfilling of the pulmonary vasculature.

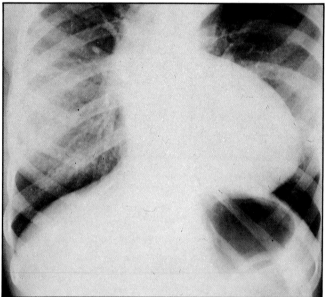

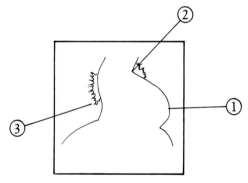

6   Chest radiograph showing right-sided aortic arch.

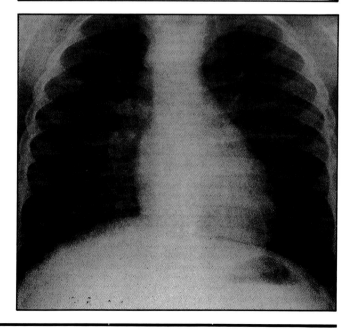

Right-Sided Aortic Arch

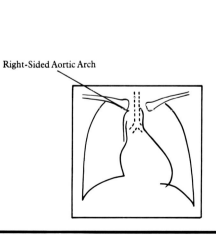

7

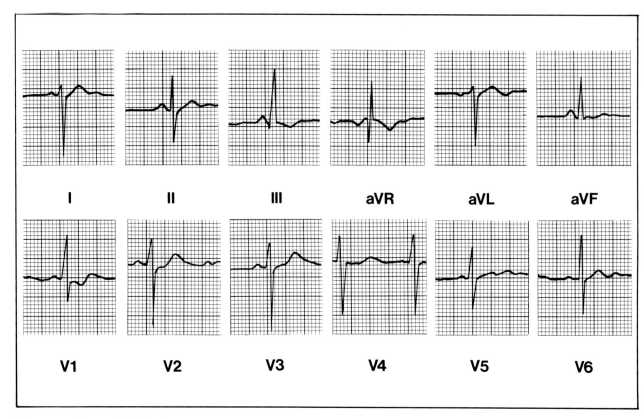

Electrocardiogram in Fallot's tetralogy showing moderate right ventricular hypertrophy.

8

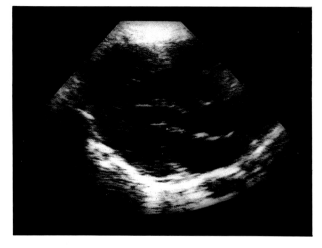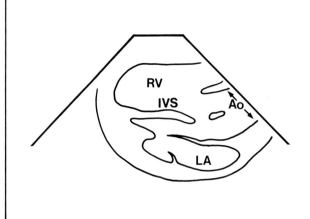

Parasternal 2-D echocardiographic long axis view showing aortic valve override of the septum. In this view the override appears to be more than 50%.

9

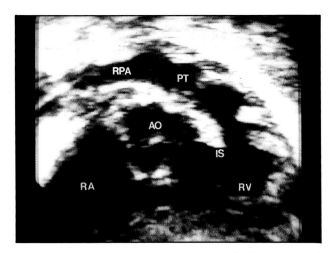

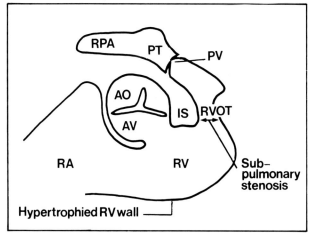

2-D echocardiographic subcostal anatomically orientated section. It shows three of the four features of Fallot's tetralogy, namely, overriding of the aortic valve, sub-pulmonary infundibular stenosis and right ventricular hypertrophy. The aorta overrides the ventricular septal defect (the fourth feature of tetralogy) not seen in this projection.

FALLOT'S TETRALOGY

Cardiac Catheterization & Angiography

10 Right ventriculogram (lateral projection) showing right-to-left shunt across the ventricular septal defect.

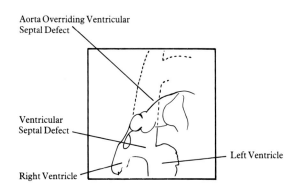

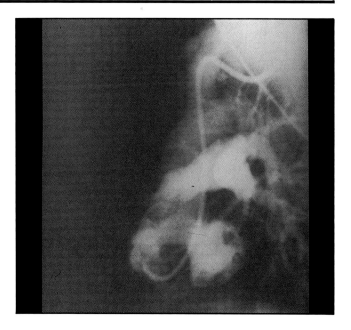

11 Right ventricular angiogram (antero-posterior projection) showing infundibular stenosis with aortic override.

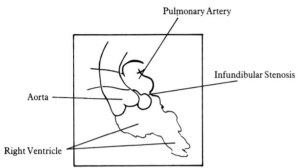

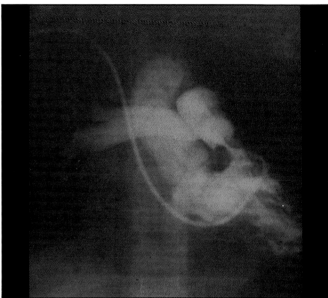

Pathology

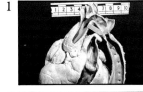

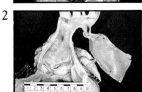

Coarctation of the aorta is a congenital constriction or narrowing of the aortic arch or descending aorta. It is of variable position, extent and severity and may be associated with other congenital abnormalities such as bicuspid aortic valve. Acquired coarctation of the aorta occurs at variable and multiple sites (Takayasu disease).

When coarctation of the aorta presents in adult life the lesion is usually a sharply localized constriction just beyond the origin of the left subclavian artery and proximal to the insertion of the ligamentum arteriosum [1]. In less than 10% of cases the coarctation extends over several centimetres. An associated bicuspid aortic valve is present in about 85% of cases [2]. In the presence of isolated coarctation a collateral circulation usually develops between the upper and lower parts of the body [3].

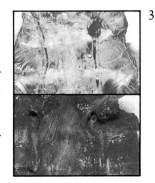

Presentation

Symptoms

Usually adults presenting with coarctation have no symptoms. The lesion is discovered at routine examination when hypertension is found or a murmur is heard. Occasionally patients present with complications eg. angina, endocarditis, myocardial infarction or dissection of the aorta. Cerebrovascular complications are not infrequent and are usually due to cerebral haemorrhage often with rupture of a berry aneurysm.

Signs

The blood pressure is usually elevated. The pulses in the legs are often weak and the femoral pulse delayed by comparison with the right brachial pulse. Prominent arterial pulsation in the suprasternal notch may be present. The development of the collateral circulation between the upper and lower parts of the body may be revealed by palpating arterial pulsations around the scapulae. The left ventricle becomes hypertrophied in response to hypertension and this may be clinically obvious on palpation with a double apical impulse. A classical auscultatory finding is an ejection systolic murmur arising at the site of the coarctation which may be best heard high up on the back over the spine. This murmur is delayed relative to an aortic valve ejection murmur and consequently appears to spill through the aortic valve closure sound. Additional auscultatory findings may be due to a coexistent bicuspid aortic valve with an ejection sound and an ejection systolic murmur. Other murmurs may be produced by turbulent blood flow in the dilated and anastomotic arteries around the scapulae. These also sound like delayed ejection or sometimes continuous murmurs.

Investigations

Radiology

The characteristic features in the chest radiograph of a discrete

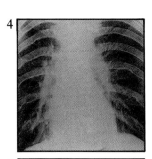

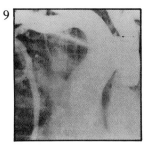

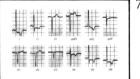

coarctation are rib notching [4], abnormalities of the aortic knuckle [5] and cardiac enlargement [6]. Rib notching is usually seen after puberty. The aortic knuckle may be flat, high or low or more rarely double. Post-stenotic dilatation of the descending aorta is a common feature.

Electrocardiography

The electrocardiogram in coarctation may be normal or show features of left ventricular hypertrophy with ST-T abnormalities in the left ventricular leads [7].

Echocardiography

The 2-dimensional echocardiogram can provide a qualitative if not quantitative assessment of the lesion from the suprasternal notch [8]. The severity of the coarctation is more readily determined by abnormalities of the left ventricle, notably hypertrophy, which can be detected by echocardiography. Another use of echocardiography is to identify the frequently associated intracardiac malformations.

Cardiac Catheterization and Angiography

There will be a systolic pressure difference between the region above the site of coarctation and the region below. The aortogram of a typical discrete coarctation shows a shelf-like narrowing at the junction between the isthmus and descending aorta [9]. With long standing severe coarctation there is visible dilatation of the internal mammary and other collateral arteries.

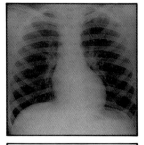

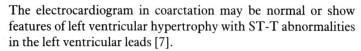

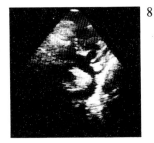

COARCTATION OF THE AORTA

1 Arch arteries showing coarctation of the aorta (arrow) just beyond the left subclavian artery. The orifices of the intercostal arteries in the descending aorta are greatly enlarged.

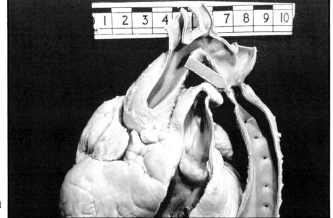

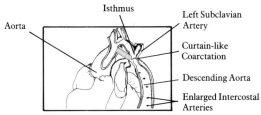

2 Arch arteries showing coarctation of the aorta with dilatation of the ascending aorta and bicuspid aortic valve.

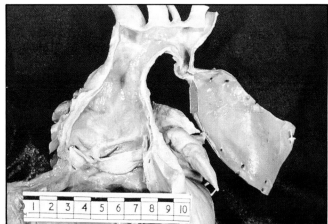

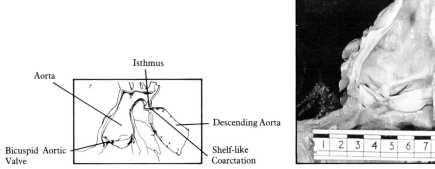

3 Panels showing the internal mammary arteries from a normal patient and a patient with coarctation. The patient with coarctation has gross dilatation of the arteries due to collateral flow.

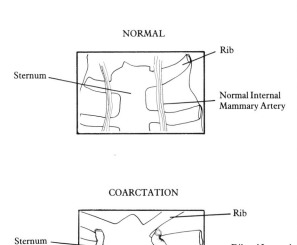

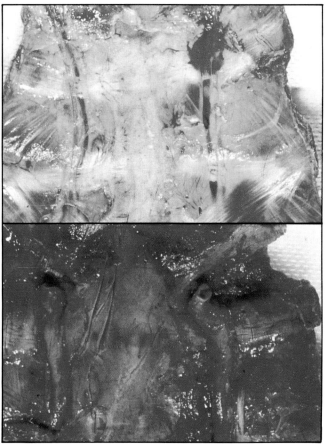

4   Chest radiograph in coarctation showing marked rib notching.

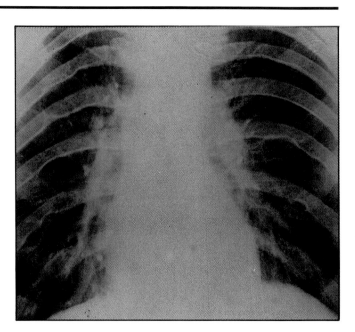

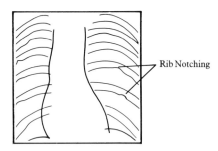

Rib Notching

5   Chest radiograph in coarctation showing a flat aortic knuckle and rib notching.

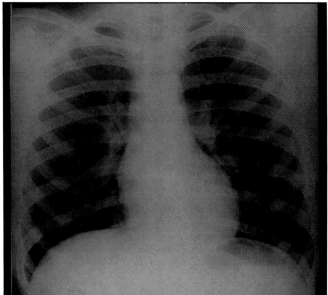

Flat Knuckle

Rib Notching

6   Chest radiograph in coarctation showing a large heart with left atrial and upper lobe vessel dilatation which indicates pulmonary venous hypertension.

Upper Lobe Vessel Dilatation

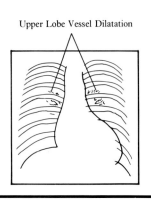

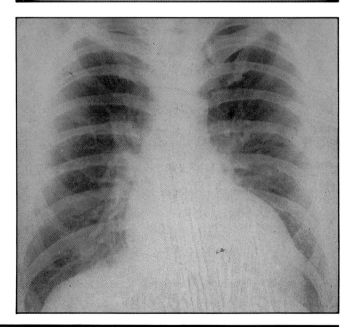

Chapter 6.

Myocardial and Pericardial Disease

Abbreviations

a	Anterior	LA	Left Atrium	Per	Pericardium
A	Atrium	LV	Left Ventricle	PVW	Posterior Ventricular
AVL	Aortic Valve Leaflet	LVEDP	Left Ventricular End		Wall
CW	Chest Wall		Diastolic Pressure	RA	Right Atrium
Eff	Effusion	MV	Mitral Valve	RV	Right Ventricle
En	Endocardium	MVL	Mitral Valve Leaflet	RVEDP	Right Ventricular End
Ep	Epicardium	p	Posterior		Diastolic Pressure
IVS	Intraventricular Septum	PE	Pericardial Effusion		

Pathology

Dilated cardiomyopathy represents end stage left ventricular muscle disease with failure of emptying in systole not due to coronary artery disease or systemic hypertension. A number of aetiological factors have been associated with the development of a dilated cardiomyopathy such as alcohol or following a viral infection, but usually no clear aetiology can be determined. The pathological features are a dilated, globular, thin walled left ventricle with a large cavity [1]. Mural thrombus frequently develops in the ventricles. Histological examination of virtually all forms of dilated cardiomyopathy reveals interstitial fibrosis and vacuolated muscle fibres [2].

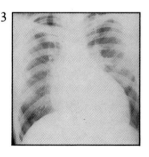

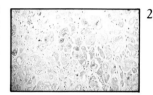

Presentation

Symptoms

Patients with dilated cardiomyopathy may be asymptomatic and present with cardiomegaly on routine chest x-ray. The symptoms include breathlessness and fatigue or even frank fluid retention due to heart failure. Occasionally, presentation is the result of systemic emboli, perhaps with associated transient arrhythmia.

Signs

The signs are those of left ventricular dysfunction with a double apical impulse and gallop rhythm on auscultation. Sinus tachycardia is common with a small, sharp upstroke arterial pulse reflecting a low cardiac output. A pansystolic murmur due to secondary mitral or tricuspid regurgitation may be present. The jugular venous pressure may show an increased 'v' wave or systolic wave if there is additional tricuspid regurgitation. Patients with fluid retention usually show frank elevation of venous pressure.

Investigations

Radiology

In dilated cardiomyopathy the chest radiograph shows non-specific cardiac enlargement and the changes in the lungs reflect the elevation of pulmonary venous pressure [3]. These include upper lobe blood divertion, Kerley's B lines and frank pulmonary oedema.

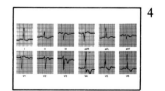

Electrocardiography

Cardiomyopathy is not associated with specific electrocardiographic abnormalities. Usually the electrocardiogram shows non-specific ST-T abnormalities [4] and sometimes left bundle branch block [5]. Some patients may show Q waves in mid precordial leads simulating myocardial infarction [6].

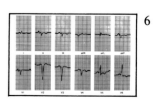

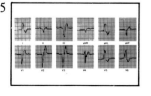

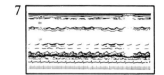

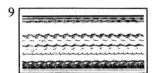

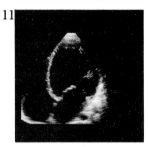

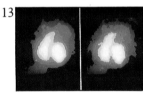

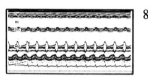

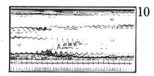

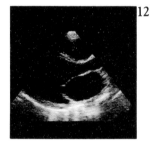

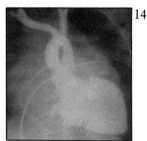

Echocardiography

The left ventricular dimensions are increased and amplitude of wall movement is reduced (i.e. reduced fractional shortening) [7]. As the stroke volume falls, the amplitude of diastolic separation of the mitral valve leaflets is reduced. A very characteristic appearance is of a low amplitude mitral echo 'floating' in a dilated ventricle [8]. Aortic root motion is also reduced so that the entire heart has a generally hypokinetic appearance [9] which is best appreciated on the slow scan from aorta to the ventricles [10], or on two-dimensional echocardiography [11,12]. Right ventricular dimension is often also increased. Slight enlargement of the left atrium due to chronic elevation of left ventricular end diastolic pressure is common.

Nuclear Techniques

Generalized abnormalities of left ventricular function may also be demonstrated using either first pass studies or gated blood pool imaging [13]. Such abnormalities may be distinguished from a left ventricular aneurysm due to coronary artery disease.

Cardiac Catheterization and Angiography

Echocardiography is so characteristic in dilated cardiomyopathy that cardiac catheterization is usually unnecessary except to exclude associated coronary artery disease. Left ventricular angiography will show a large volume left ventricle with a grossly reduced ejection fraction [14].

1   Dilated cardiomyopathy: the opened left ventricle has a large cavity and thin wall.

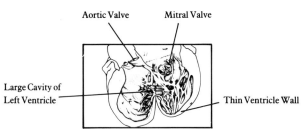

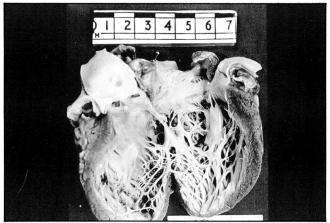

2   Histological appearance of non-specific dilated cardiomyopathy. The muscle fibres vary in size and are vacuolated. Fibrosis is increased between the muscle fibres.

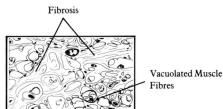

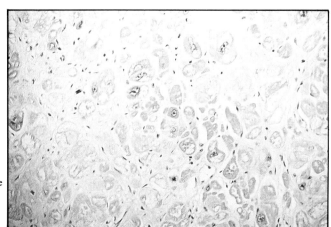

DILATED CARDIOMYOPATHY   Radiology

3   Chest radiograph in dilated cardiomyopathy showing a large heart with pulmonary venous hypertension.

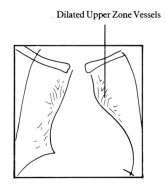

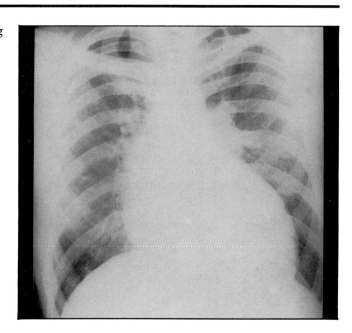

4

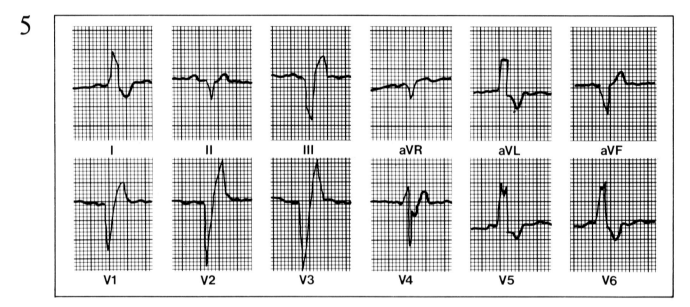

Electrocardiogram in a patient with dilated cardiomyopathy showing non-specific ST-T abnormalities.

5

Electrocardiogram in a patient with dilated cardiomyopathy showing left bundle branch block.

6

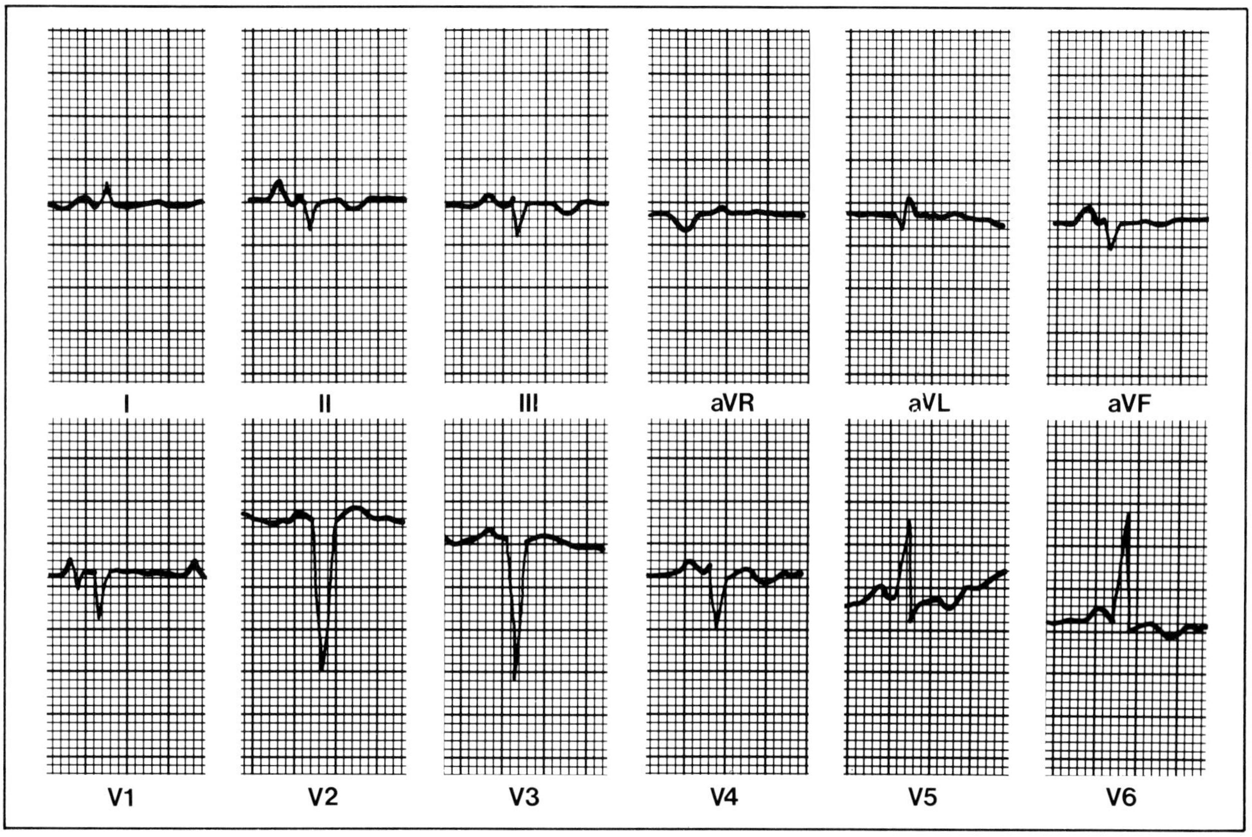

Electrocardiogram in a patient with dilated cardiomyopathy with septal Q-waves simulating myocardial infarction.

DILATED CARDIOMYOPATHY

Echocardiography

7

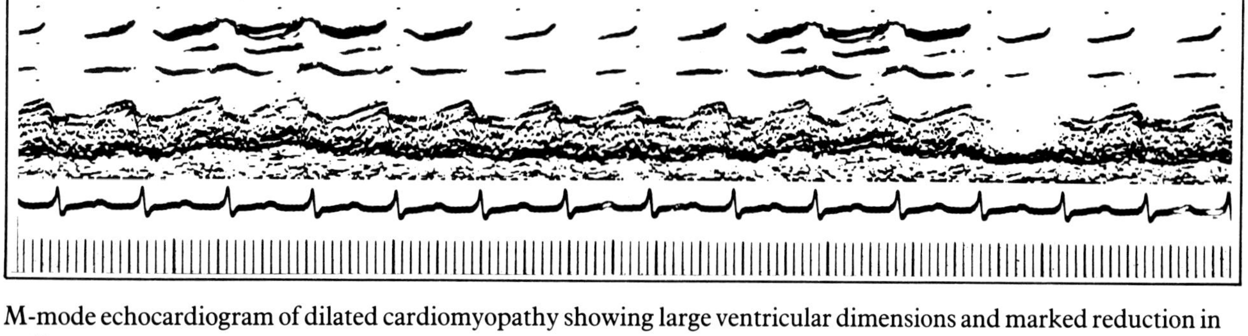

M-mode echocardiogram of dilated cardiomyopathy showing large ventricular dimensions and marked reduction in wall movement.

8

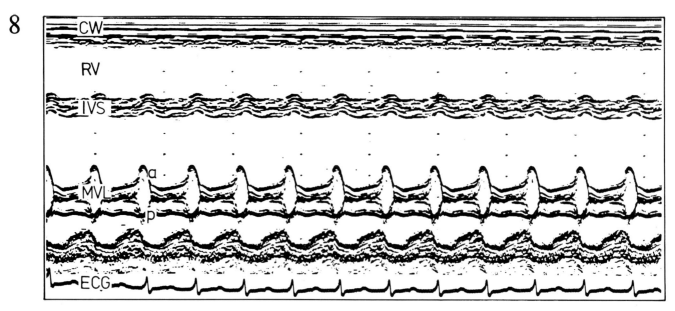

M-mode echocardiogram in dilated cardiomyopathy showing reduction in amplitude of the anterior leaflet of the mitral valve.

9

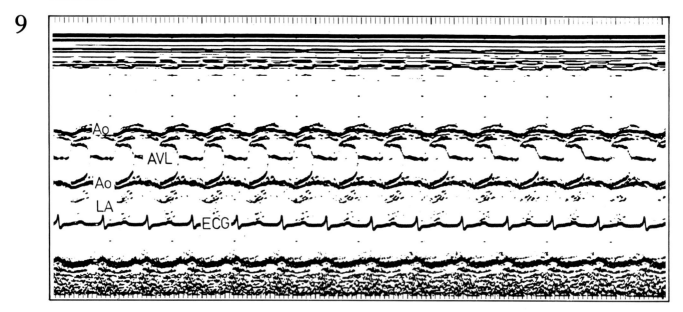

M-mode echocardiogram of dilated cardiomyopathy showing reduced aortic root motion.

10

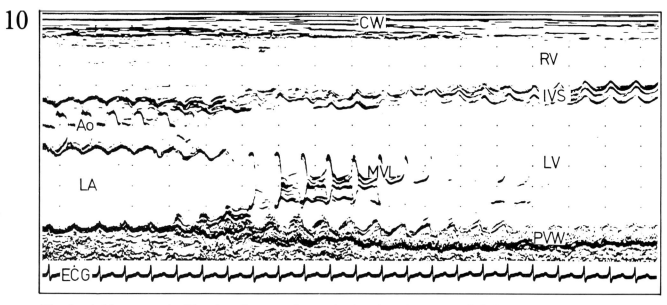

The slow left heart scan in dilated cardiomyopathy emphasises the enlargement of all chambers and the generalised hypokinesia.

11

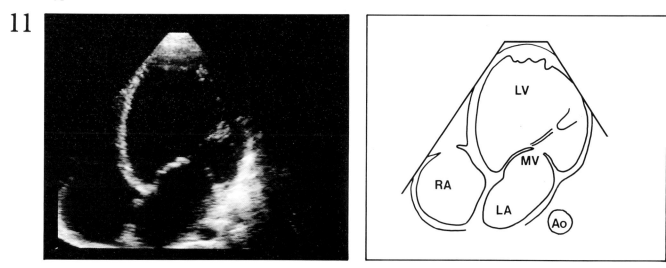

2-D echocardiographic apical four-chamber view showing left ventricular dilatation cardiomyopathy. Note the thin-walled globular left ventricle. The irregularities in the apex may be due to thrombus.

12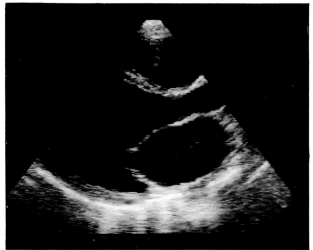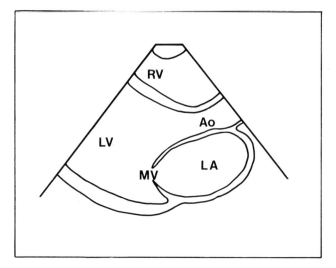

2-D echocardiographic parasternal long axis diastolic view showing left atrial and left ventricular enlargement. The small separation of the mitral valve leaflets indicates the low blood flow through the valve.

13 Gated blood pool scan showing little difference in the size of the ventricular cavities between end diastole (left) and end systole (right).

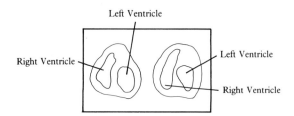 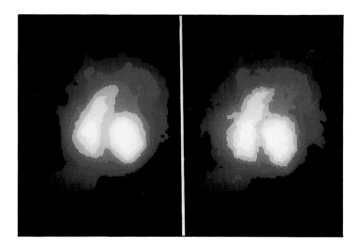

14 Left ventricular angiogram (antero-posterior projection) showing a dilated left ventricle in systole.

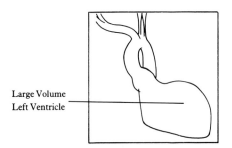

Large Volume
Left Ventricle

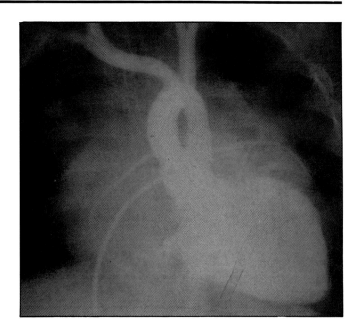

HYPERTROPHIC CARDIOMYOPATHY

Pathology

Hypertrophic cardiomyopathy is a condition in which there is hypertrophy of the left ventricle without obvious cause. This pathological process includes a spectrum ranging from a left ventricle which is concentrically hypertrophied [1] to septal hypertrophy disproportionate to the hypertrophy of the left ventricular free wall [2], or there may be localized hypertrophy of the apex of the left ventricle. Where there is asymmetrical septal hypertrophy, the septum may project into the left or right ventricles [3] or both. In cases where left ventricular obstruction occurs, a patch of endocardial thickening develops over the septum due to contact with the anterior cusp of the mitral valve [4].

Histological examination will often reveal only non-specific hypertrophied muscle bundles. Alternatively, some areas of abnormal muscle may show fibres arranged in circular whorls or in clusters with fibres radiating out from a central point [5]; examination at ultrastructural level shows myofibrillar disorganisation within individual cells.

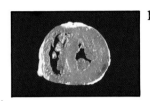
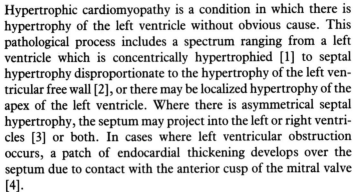
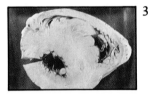
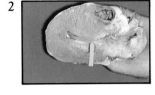
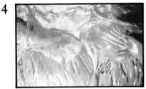
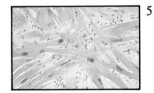

Presentation

Symptoms

There may be no symptoms and patients may present with a chance finding of left ventricular hypertrophy without an obvious cause. Patients with septal hypertrophy may also be asymptomatic and may be identified because a murmur is heard at a routine clinical examination. Symptomatic patients complain of angina, exertional syncope or dyspnoea. Tachycardia induced by exercise results in a shortening of ventricular diastole which reduces the time available for coronary filling with consequent myocardial ischaemia and angina. Myocardial ischaemia may lead to ventricular fibrillation and sudden death. Incomplete left atrial emptying during exercise tachycardia leads to a rise in left atrial and pulmonary venous pressure resulting in breathlessness. Incomplete left ventricular filling due to a tachycardia can lead to a reduction in left ventricular stroke volume and systemic hypotension which may cause syncope.

Signs

Hypertrophy of the left ventricle makes it stiff; this results in an augmented left atrial contraction which may be palpable as a separate (double) impulse and audible as a fourth heart sound. In the presence of obstruction, the carotid pulse is jerky or sharp in its upstroke. This may be due to increased velocity of contraction and the increased rate of rise of left ventricular and aortic pressures early in systole. The jugular venous pulse may show abnormal 'a' wave dominance due to enhanced right atrial contraction as a result of either generalised right ventricular hypertrophy or hypertrophy of the septum encroaching on the right ventricular cavity. The systolic murmur may be due to turbulence created in the left ventricular outflow tract or due to mitral regurgitation as the anterior cusp of the closed mitral valve moves forward to meet the bulging hypertrophied septum. In either case the murmur will be delayed in systole. The second heart sound may be split physiologically or it may be reversed due to prolongation of left ventricular systole.

Investigations

Radiology

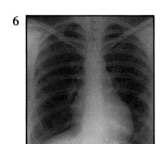

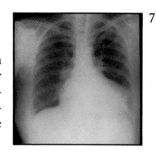

The heart is often enlarged and the diagnosis may be suggested on the chest radiograph by a slight bulge on the high left ventricular border due to septal hypertrophy [6]. In severe cases the pulmonary venous pressure may be raised; this is reflected by cardiomegaly, left atrial dilatation, and dilatation of the upper zone pulmonary vessels [7].

Electrocardiography

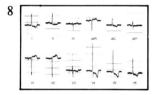

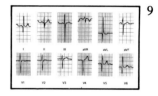

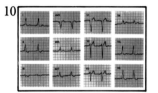

The electrocardiographic features of hypertrophic cardiomyopathy are variable. The electrocardiogram may be normal or strikingly abnormal without reflecting the severity of the pathological abnormality or haemodynamic derangement. Left ventricular hypertrophy usually with marked T wave inversion may be seen [8]. In some patients the initial Q wave in the left precordial leads is absent. Steep QR or QRS waves simulating myocardial infarction may be seen in other patients [9]. These features have been attributed to septal hypertrophy and fibrosis. Atrial fibrillation may develop in advanced cases. The PR interval may be short with features suggestive of pre-excitation (Wolff-Parkinson-White syndrome) [10]. Left bundle branch block is uncommon.

Echocardiography

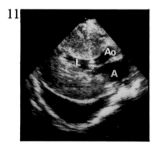

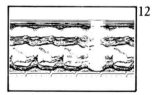

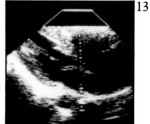

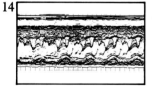

The echocardiogram permits direct visualization of the thickness of the ventricular walls and interventricular septum.

There may be concentric hypertrophy of the left ventricle [11]. Septal thickness may or may not exceed that of the free wall [12], but in many cases it is gross and it appears to obliterate the right ventricular cavity making definition of its right sided endocardial surface difficult. The left ventricular cavity is usually small and despite the immobile septum fractional shortening is normal or increased due to vigorous movement of the posterior wall. Apical hypertrophy will be visible on 2-D echocardiography [13].

Movement of the mitral valve appears to be restricted by the small ventricular cavity and the anterior leaflet appears to hit the ventricular septum as it opens in diastole [14]. A characteristic part of the mitral valve echo is the so called 'systolic anterior movement' (SAM). Soon after mitral valve closure, a group of echoes moves forwards from the closure line towards the septum, the anterior of which comes to close approximation to the septal endocardium. At the end of systole the echoes return to the closure line.

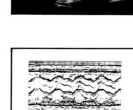

At the onset of ventricular ejection the aortic valve opens normally. If obstruction develops in mid systole the valve leaflets show a coarse fluttering motion and begin to come together [15].

Finally, complete closure of the valve occurs at the normal time or is even delayed if left ventricular ejection is prolonged.

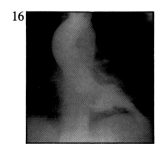

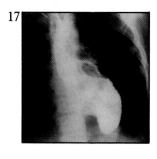

Cardiac Catheterization and Angiography

The characteristic haemodynamic abnormality is an elevation of left ventricular end-diastolic pressure due to the stiffness of the left ventricle. The presence of obstruction may be detected either as a resting systolic pressure difference between the cavity and outflow portion of the left ventricle or as a result of various manoeuvres which reduce left ventricular cavity size (e.g. amyl nitrate or Valsalva manoeuvre). In contrast to aortic valve stenosis, following a premature ventricular beat aortic pressure may fall while left ventricular systolic pressure increases; this either results in an augmented pressure difference or the development of a pressure difference if none was present at rest.

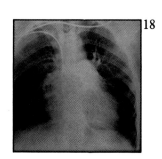

Left ventricular angiography shows a small cavity, apical obliteration and prominent papillary muscles [16,17]. The ventricle often has an irregular outline and there may be mitral regurgitation. Right ventricular angiography may show infundibular obstruction due to septal hypertrophy [18].

1 Transverse section through the heart in cardiomyopathy showing concentric left ventricular hypertrophy.

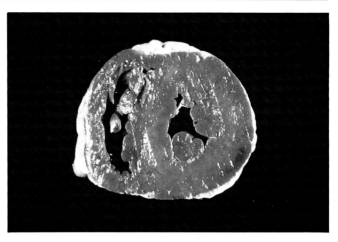

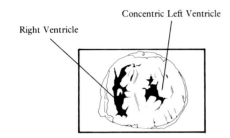

2 The left ventricle from a patient with hypertrophic cardiomyopathy showing a small cavity with very thick wall. The septal region is asymmetrically thickened being at least twice as thick as the parietal wall. The septum bulges into the outflow tract of the left ventricle and impinges onto the anterior cusp of the mitral valve (arrow).

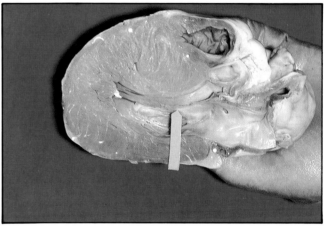

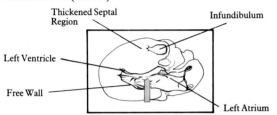

3 Transverse section across the left and right ventricles in hypertrophic cardiomyopathy. The septum is approximately two and a half times the thickness of the left ventricular free wall and bulges into the right ventricular outflow tract.

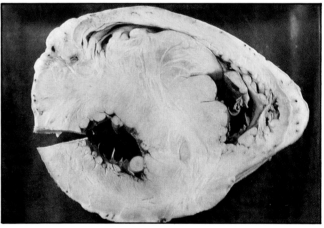

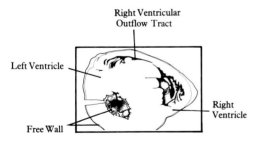

4 Pathological specimen showing thickening of the anterior leaflet of the mitral valve with a corresponding thickening on the ventricular septum opposite (arrowed), indicating contact in life with an obstruction to ventricular outflow.

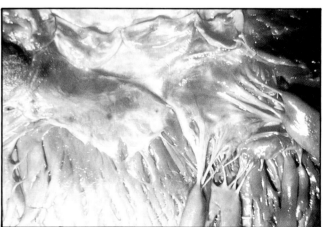

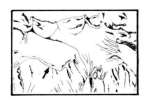

HYPERTROPHIC CARDIOMYOPATHY Pathology／Radiology

5   Histological section of the myocardium in hypertrophic cardiomyopathy. The muscle fibres are
arranged in a characteristic cross-over pattern radiating out in all directions rather than being arranged in
parallel fashion.

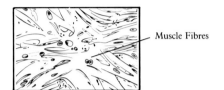

Muscle Fibres

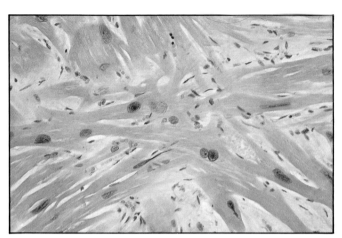

HYPERTROPHIC CARDIOMYOPATHY Radiology

6   Chest radiograph showing large heart with bulge on
high left ventricular border characteristic of septal
hypertrophy.

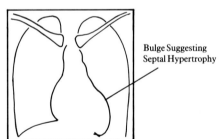

Bulge Suggesting
Septal Hypertrophy

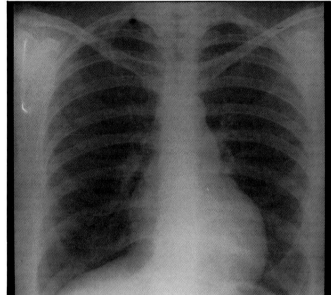

7 Chest radiograph showing large heart and left atrium with pulmonary venous hypertension.

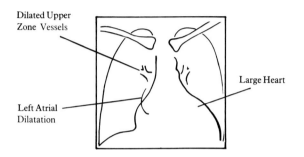

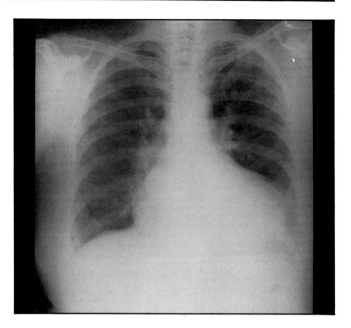

HYPERTROPHIC CARDIOMYOPATHY

Electrocardiography

8

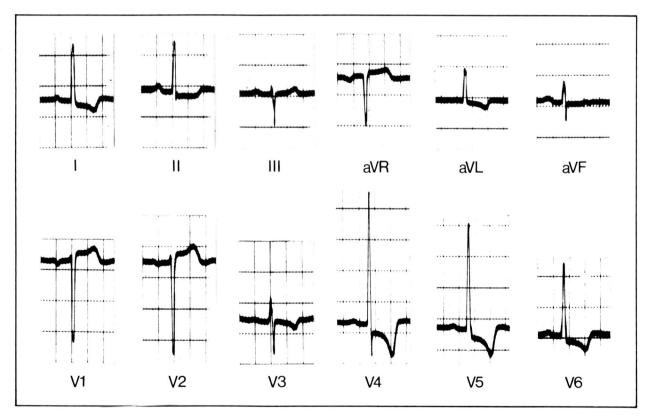

Electrocardiogram of a patient with hypertrophic cardiomyopathy. Note high voltage in chest leads and T-wave inversion in left ventricular leads. All chest leads 1mV=0.5cm.

9

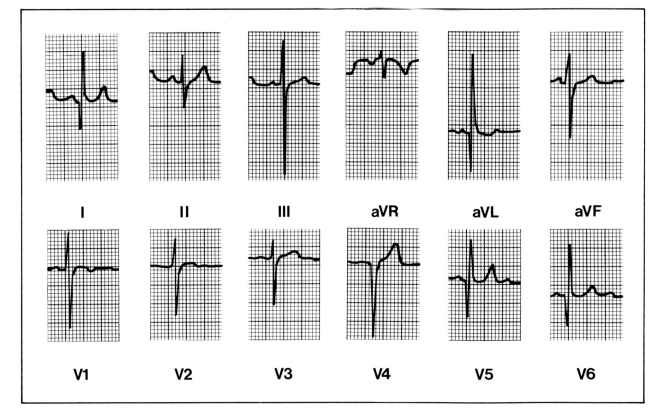

Electrocardiogram of a patient with hypertrophic cardiomyopathy, showing well developed Q-waves in lead 1, aVL and V4 to V6, simulating myocardial infarction.

10

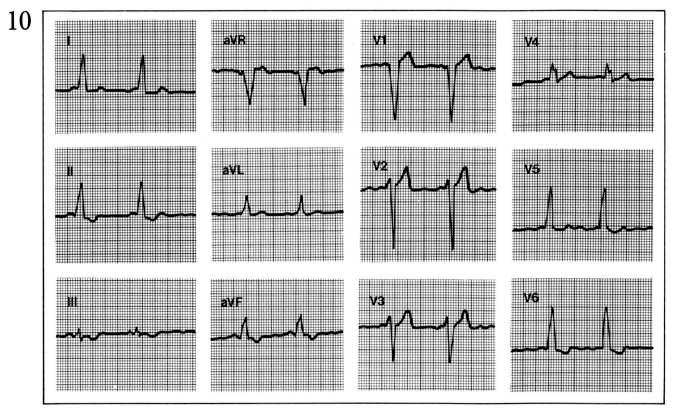

Electrocardiogram showing shortening of the PR interval, widening of the QRS complex and a delta wave indicative of pre-excitation. This is an occasional feature of hypertrophic cardiomyopathy.

11

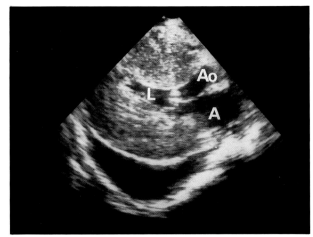
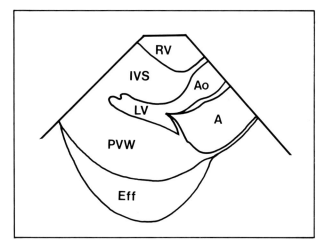

2-D echocardiographic parasternal long axis systolic view in hypertrophic cardiomyopathy with gross symmetrical hypertrophy of the left ventricle with slit-like cavity. Note additional pericardial effusion.

12

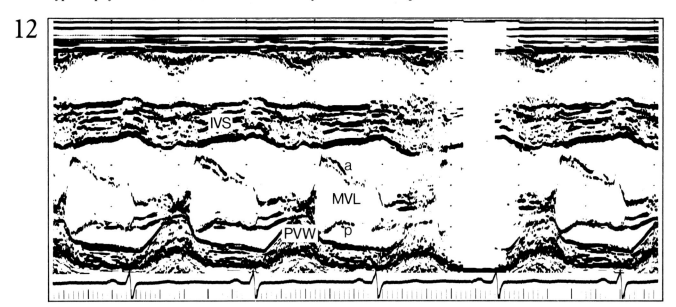

M-mode echocardiogram of mild hypertrophic cardiomyopathy. The only abnormality is that the septum is thicker than the posterior left ventricular wall.

13

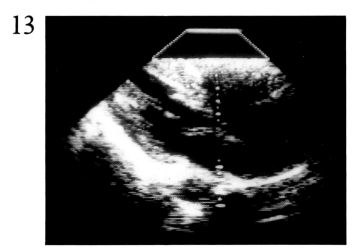
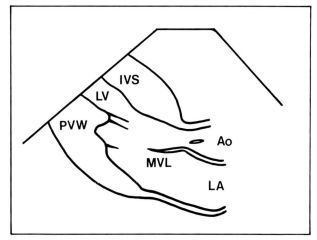

2-D echocardiographic parasternal long axis view showing hypertrophy, particularly in the apical region.

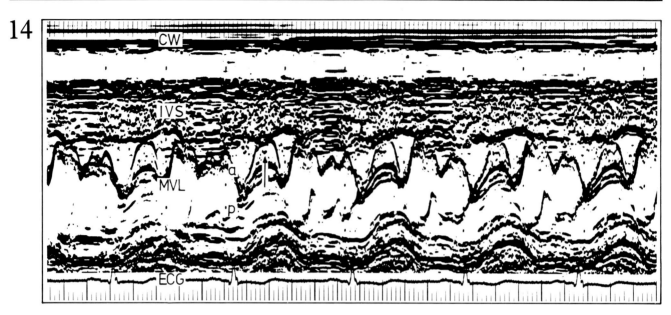

M-mode echocardiogram of hypertrophic cardiomyopathy with left ventricular outflow obstruction. The echocardiogram shows systolic anterior movement of the anterior leaflet (arrowed) which also strikes the septum at the onset of diastole.

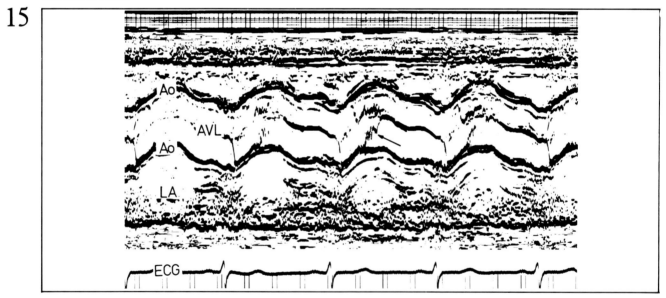

M-mode echocardiogram of the aortic valve showing mid-systolic closure and fluttering (arrowed). This may be seen in hypertrophic cardiomyopathy but it is a non-specific feature.

16 Left ventricular angiogram in systole (antero-posterior projection) showing a small irregular cavity.

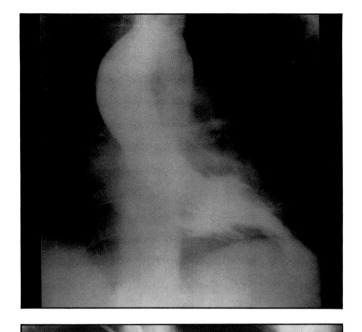

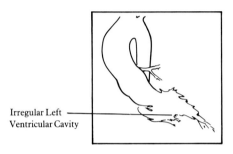

Irregular Left
Ventricular Cavity

17 Left ventricular angiogram in diastole (antero-posterior projection) showing an irregular outline and inferior indentation from asymmetric septal hypertrophy.

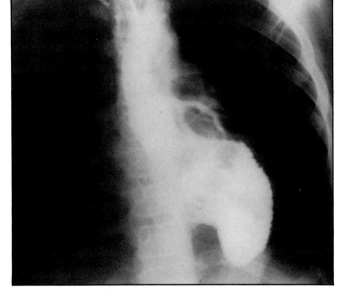

Aorta

Hypertrophied
Septum

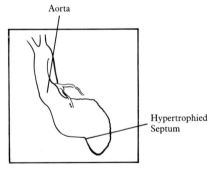

18 Right ventricular angiogram (antero-posterior projection) showing infundibular obstruction due to septal hypertrophy.

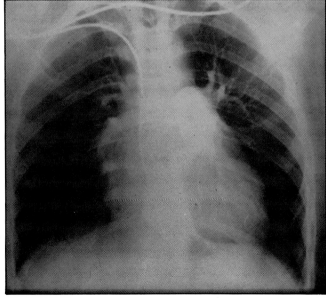

Pulmonary Artery

Septal Hypertrophy

Right Ventricle

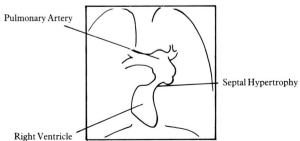

Pathology

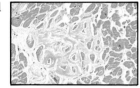

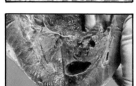

Restrictive cardiomyopathy is characterized by a restriction to diastolic filling and ventricular distensibility which can be brought about by endocardial and/or myocardial lesions. Signs of 'heart failure' which result are not related to abnormal systolic myocardial function but are the result of back pressure due to impaired diastolic filling. When this process becomes extensive, often due to super-added thrombus on top of endocardial scarring, the already small ventricular cavity may become 'obliterated'. Systolic function is usually well preserved.

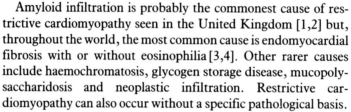

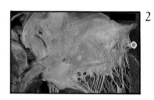

Amyloid infiltration is probably the commonest cause of restrictive cardiomyopathy seen in the United Kingdom [1,2] but, throughout the world, the most common cause is endomyocardial fibrosis with or without eosinophilia [3,4]. Other rarer causes include haemochromatosis, glycogen storage disease, mucopolysaccharidosis and neoplastic infiltration. Restrictive cardiomyopathy can also occur without a specific pathological basis.

Presentation

Symptoms

Patients usually present with dyspnoea, ankle and abdominal swelling. There may be marked fluid retention while paroxysmal nocturnal dyspnoea or orthopnoea are absent. Although the reasons are not known, ascites may be much more marked than peripheral oedema. Occasionally patients may present with palpitations due to atrial or ventricular arrhythmias. They may present with syncope due to conducting tissue involvement. Orthostatic hypotension may occur due to over-dehydration with diuretics, or due to amyloid infiltration of the autonomic nervous system.

Signs

Physical examination reveals evidence of restrictive filling of the right ventricle with an elevated jugular venous pressure, which may be further elevated by deep inspiration (Kussmaul's sign), peripheral oedema and ascites. The liver is often enlarged. There may be signs of a low cardiac output. Auscultation often reveals a gallop rhythm and systolic murmurs due to atrio-ventricular valvular regurgitation.

Investigations

Radiology

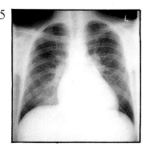

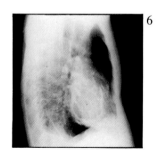

The chest x-ray is generally unremarkable but there may be cardiomegaly usually due to bi-atrial dilatation [5]. Pulmonary oedema may be present particularly when mitral regurgitation, due to tethering of the posterior leaflet of the mitral valve is the main haemodynamic lesion.

Pericardial calcification is absent in restrictive cardiomyopathy and when present enables the diagnosis of constrictive pericarditis to be made [6]. The distinction between the two conditions is a common problem in differential diagnosis.

Electrocardiography

The electrocardiogram may show sinus rhythm, supraventricular arrhythmias (usually atrial fibrillation), or heart block due to conducting tissue involvement by fibrosis. Low voltage may be seen particularly in the presence of an accompanying pericardial effusion. ST-segment depression and T-wave inversion changes (in the absence of voltage criteria of left ventricular hypertrophy) may be seen and are thought to be due to myocardial fibrosis.

Echocardiography

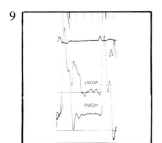

M-mode echocardiography reveals non-specific changes, including right ventricular dilatation with a normal-sized or small left ventricle [7]. Two-dimensional echocardiography is extremely helpful in the early diagnosis of restrictive cardiomyopathy and specific cavity changes such as apical obliteration and endocardial thickening can be easily demonstrated. Amyloid infiltration gives a particular and diagnostic reflection pattern on grey scale and this can be further characterised by amplitude processed colour-coded tissue characterisation techniques [8]. A highly specific feature of endomyocardial fibrosis well seen on the long axis 2-dimensional view is that of tethering of the posterior mitral valve leaflet.

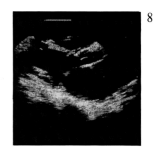

Cardiac Catheterization and Angiography

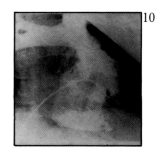

Catheterization reveals elevated ventricular filling pressures in both right and left ventricles and the filling pressures in the two ventricles differ with higher pressure in the left ventricle, unlike constrictive pericarditis where the pressures are usually equal. A prominent early diastolic dip and mid-late diastolic plateau is characteristically noted in both ventricular pressure pulses [9].

If the aetiology is endomyocardial fibrosis left ventricular angiography frequently reveals cavity obliteration and mitral regurgitation. Left ventricular systolic function is generally intact and right ventricular angiography shows tricuspid regurgitation and right ventricular apical cavity obliteration [10]. The coronary arteries are normal. If the aetiology is amyloid, left ventricular systolic function may be normal or slightly impaired, while the right ventricular cavity is dilated with tricuspid regurgitation. Endomyocardial biopsy will be needed to confirm the diagnosis histologically.

1 Amyloid deposition in the myocardium. In haematoxylin and eosin stained histological sections amyloid is a pale pink homogenous material. Amyloid [arrows] is laid down between myocardial cells and ultimately completely surrounds them leaving a lattice of amyloid within which are embedded a few residual muscle cells staining a deeper pink colour.

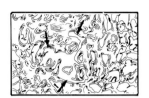

2 Macroscopic view of heart with cardiac amyloid showing amyloid deposits in the left atrium. After fixation in formalin, inspection of the surface of the left atrium shows deposits of amyloid as brown translucent nodules, 1–2 mm in diameter, just beneath the endocardium. Similar deposits are present in this specimen within the posterior cusp of the mitral valve but not in the anterior cusp.

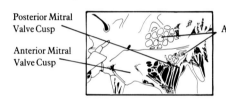

Posterior Mitral Valve Cusp
Anterior Mitral Valve Cusp
Amyloid Deposits

3 Section through the left ventricle in endomyocardial fibrosis. There is marked left ventricular apical obliteration with endocardial thickening and super-added thrombus.

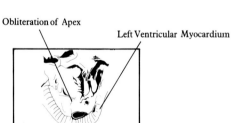

Obliteration of Apex
Left Ventricular Myocardium

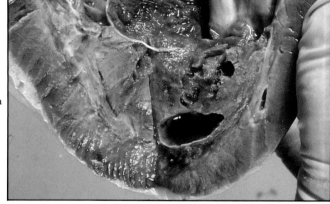

4 Endomyocardial fibrosis. The endocardium is markedly thickened and using haematoxylin and eosin (left hand panel) it is not easy to distinguish the cause of this thickening. However staining by a trichrome method (right panel) reveals that the endocardial thickening is due to a deep layer of collagen, staining blue, and a more superficial layer of fibrin.

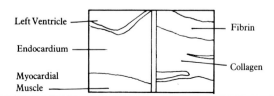

Left Ventricle
Endocardium
Myocardial Muscle
Fibrin
Collagen

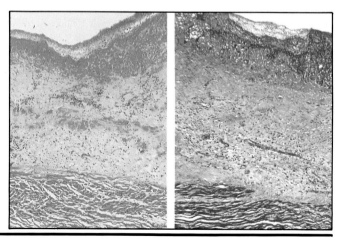

5   Chest radiograph showing cardiomegaly due to bi-atrial enlargement.

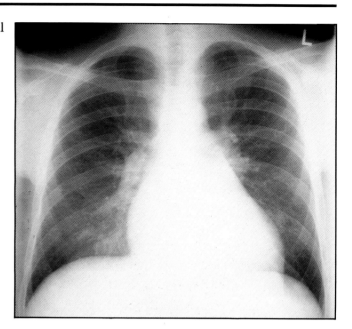

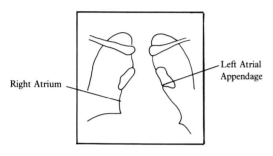

6   Lateral chest radiograph showing marked pericardial calcification.

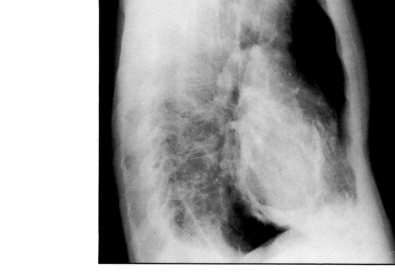

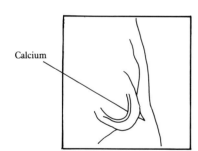

7

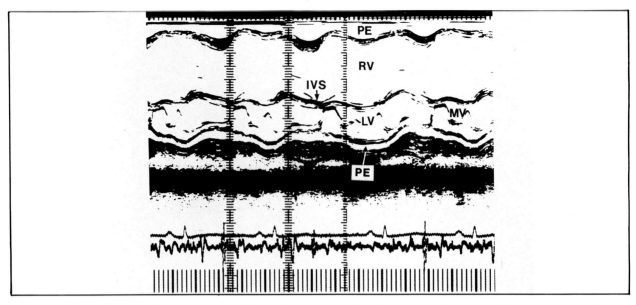

M-mode echocardiogram of endomyocardial fibrosis showing a dilated right ventricle, a small left ventricle and a pericardial effusion.

8

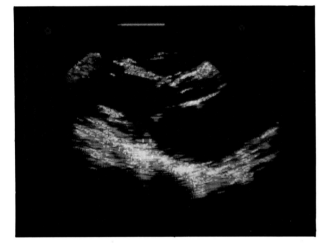 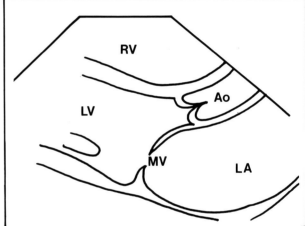

2-D echocardiographic amplitude process colour-coded long axis parasternal view in endomyocardial fibrosis showing increased echo density and endocardial thickening on the posterior left ventricular wall, thickening and tethering of the posterior mitral valve leaflet and left atrial cavity dilatation.

9 Pressure recordings taken from the right and left
ventricles simultaneously in endomyocardial fibrosis
showing the typical 'dip and plateau' and the elevated
and *different* end diastolic pressure measurements.

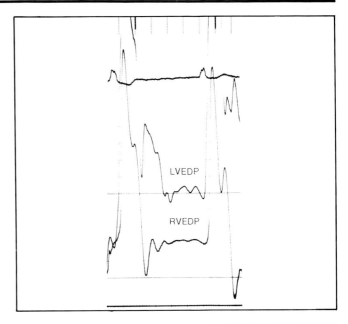

10 Right ventricular angiogram showing apical cavity
obliteration and tricuspid regurgitation due to
endomyocardial fibrosis.

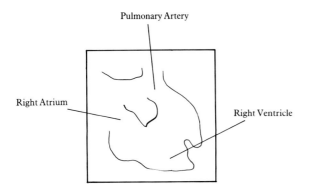

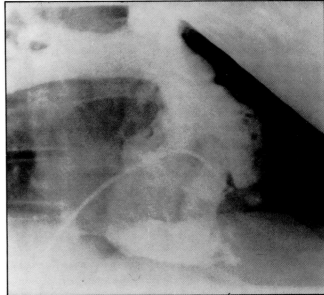

Pathology

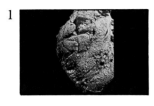

Acute pericarditis is characterised by a fibrinous exudate [1] over the visceral and parietal pericardium with varying amounts of rather turbid yellow fluid found in the pericardial cavity. Histological examination shows strands of fibrin deposited on the serosa with dilated blood vessels and an acute inflammatory infiltrate.

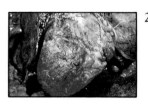

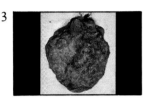

The commonest causes of acute pericarditis are viral infection [2] and acute myocardial infarction. The pericardial reaction is non-specific, although clinical data usually allows the causes to be distinguished. Viral (Coxsackie) pericarditis in fatal cases is usually associated with myocarditis. Rarely bacterial infection of the pericardium gives rise to purulent pericarditis [3].

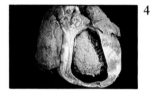

Chronic fibrosing constrictive pericarditis is usually due to tuberculosis [4]. The typical histology of giant cell granulomata may be found. However, many cases of constrictive pericarditis are due to a simple sheet of fibrous tissue in which a few lymphocytic foci are present [5]. The aetiology cannot be established: some may be due to rheumatoid disease, some to organisation of uraemic pericarditis. The majority are assumed to be post-viral.

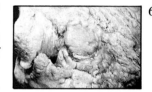

Secondary carcinoma commonly involves the pericardium [6]. The tumour may appear as white nodules over the visceral pericardium or as a more diffuse sheet of tumour.

Presentation

Symptoms

The presenting symptom of acute pericarditis is stabbing chest pain that is characteristically worse on movement. It should be distinguished from pleuritic chest pain but the distinction may be difficult. Fever and malaise are common accompaniments. Severe breathlessness may suggest the development of cardiac tamponade.

In long standing constrictive pericarditis patients may complain of abdominal distention and peripheral oedema due to the high venous pressure.

Signs

The hallmark of acute pericarditis is a pericardial rub, but this may come and go. With the accumulation of pericardial fluid, signs of tamponade may occur. On inspiration there is a marked fall in systolic blood pressure (pulsus paradoxus) and a rise in venous pressure with a dominant systolic descent. A third heart sound will not be heard.

In chronic constrictive pericarditis the physical signs will be the same as with tamponade unless the disease process has significantly involved the myocardium. Myocardial involvement is distinguished by diastolic collapse in the venous pressure and the presence of a third heart sound. Hepatomegaly, ascites and peripheral oedema may be present.

Investigations

Radiology

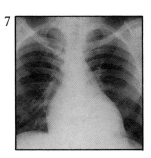

In acute pericarditis in which there is no effusion, the chest x-ray will be normal. Non-specific enlargement of the cardiac silhouette will be seen if the pericardial effusion is sufficiently large [7].

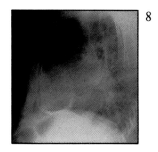

Constrictive pericarditis is calcified in approximately 50% of cases. The calcification is most commonly confined to the atrioventricular groove as seen in the penetrated and lateral chest x-rays [8]. Often, however, no abnormality is seen on the chest x-ray even though constriction is present.

Electrocardiography

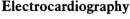

The electrocardiogram in pericardial disease usually shows non-specific ST-T abnormalities. Typically there is concave ST elevation in the acute phase [9] while T-wave inversion occurs later [10].

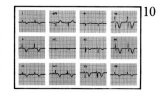

Echocardiography

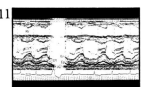

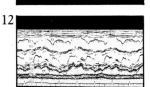

Echocardiography is the most reliable and sensitive method for making the diagnosis of a pericardial effusion. Some broad classification of the size of a pericardial effusion is possible from M mode studies. Normally visceral and parietal pericardial layers are in apposition and posteriorly return a single dense echo which moves with the endocardial echo. In pericardial effusion the two pericardial layers are separated by the fluid with the visceral pericardium moving normally with the posterior left ventricular wall, and the parietal layer immobile and separated from it by an echo free space [11]. Most frequently an echo free space can be visualised posteriorly. However, when fluid is present anteriorly, a space between the static chest wall echoes and those from the mobile right ventricular anterior wall may be observed [12]. With small amounts of fluid the gap is seen in systole, but with larger collections it is apparent throughout the cardiac cycle.

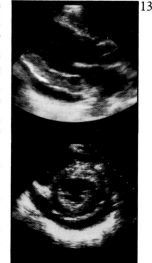

The extent and distribution of fluid surrounding the heart are much better assessed by 2-dimensional echocardiography [13]. The heart may take on a characteristic swinging motion within the bag of fluid if the effusion is large.

There are no diagnostic echocardiographic features of chronic pericardial disease without effusion. Even if calcification is present it cannot be visualised.

Cardiac Catheterization and Angiography

Cardiac catheterization and angiocardiography play little part in the diagnosis or management of patients with pericardial disease. If constriction or tamponade is present then the diastolic pressures in all the cardiac chambers will be equal. A characteristic dip and plateau is seen in the diastolic pressure but in contrast to restrictive cardiomyopathy the diastolic pressure in the two ventricles are the same.

1 Acute pericarditis. A thick fibrinous exudate covers the surface of the heart.

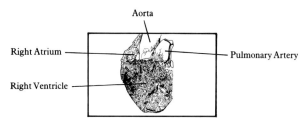

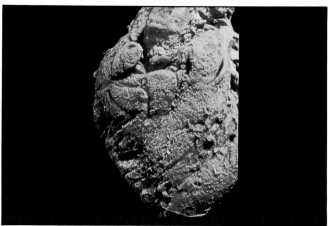

2 Viral pericarditis. The visceral pericardium is red and inflamed with a roughened surface due to deposition of fibrin.

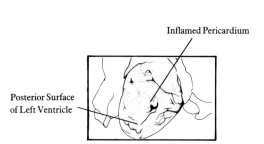

3 Bacterial pericarditis. Purulent exudate on visceral pericardium.

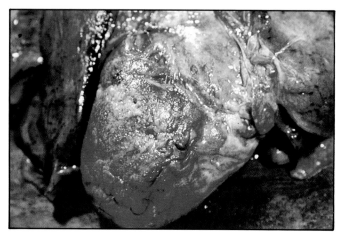

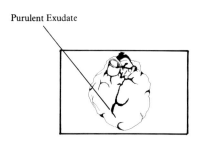

4 Chronic constrictive pericarditis. A window has been cut through the thickened parietal pericardium which forms a rough constrictive membrane. Note also the shaggy exudate on the visceral pericardium.

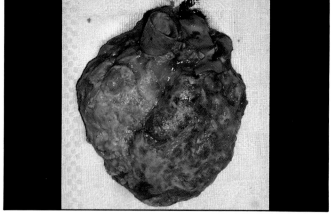

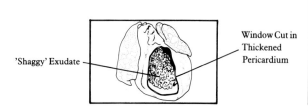

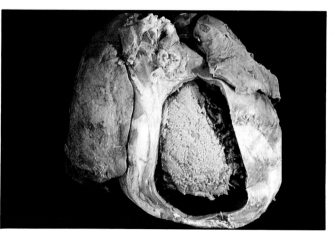

5 Histological section of normal pericardium [left]. The pericardium forms a thin layer on the myocardium. Histological section of grossly thickened pericardium [right] in chronic constrictive pericarditis. (Both sections are taken at the same magnification.)

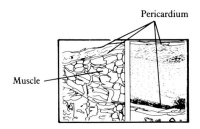

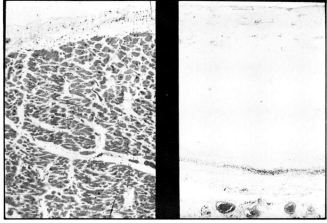

6 Secondary pericardial tumour. The pericardial cavity is opened to show the wide dissemination of tumour on the visceral pericardium of the right ventricle.

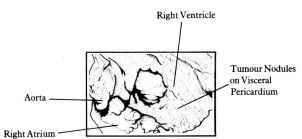

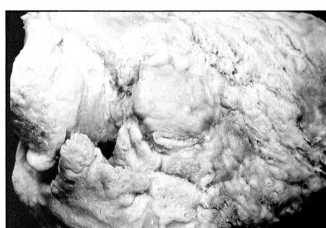

7 Chest radiography showing non-specific cardiac enlargement in pericardial effusion.

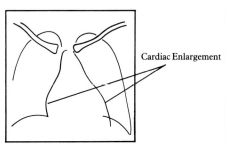

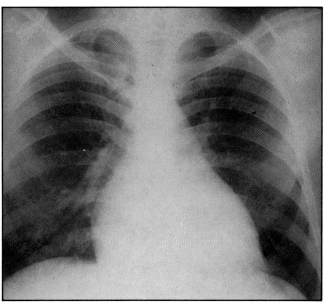

8   Lateral chest x-ray showing calcification in the atrioventricular groove in a patient with chronic constrictive pericarditis.

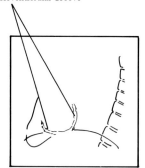

Calcification in Atrioventricular Groove

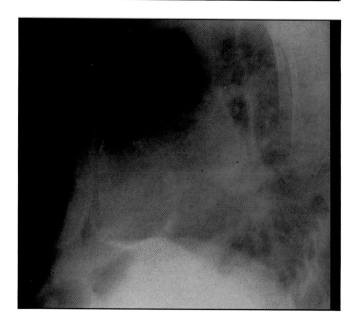

PERICARDIAL DISEASE

Electrocardiography

9

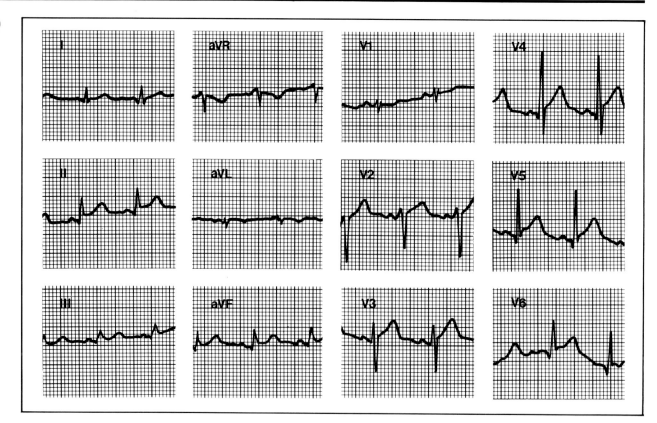

Electrocardiogram showing widespread concave ST-segment elevation in a patient with acute pericarditis.

10

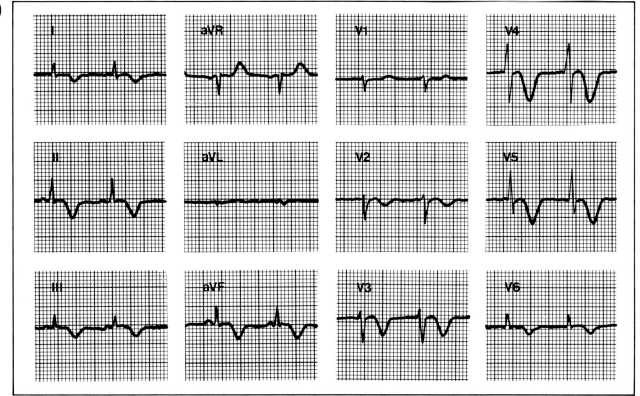

Electrocardiogram showing widespread T-wave inversion following acute pericarditis.

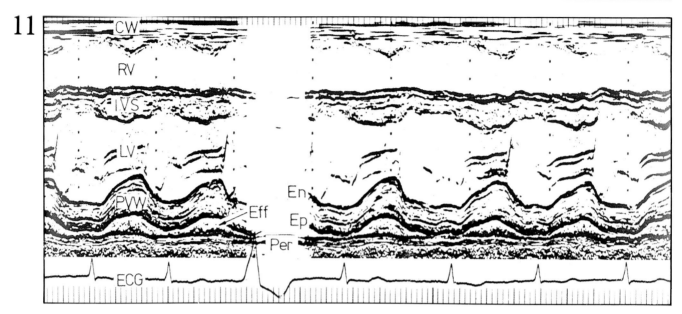

M-mode echocardiogram showing small posterior pericardial effusion. The parietal pericardial layer is immobile while the visceral layer moves with the posterior left ventricular endocardium

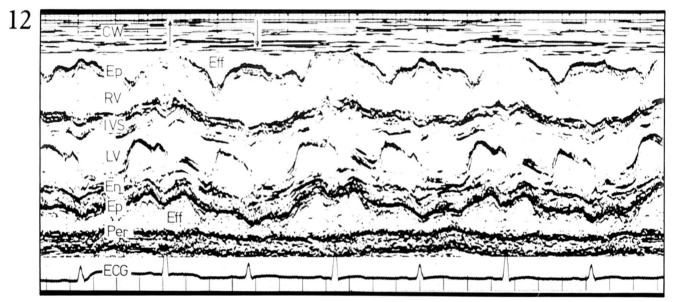

M-mode echocardiogram showing both anterior and posterior pericardial effusion.

13

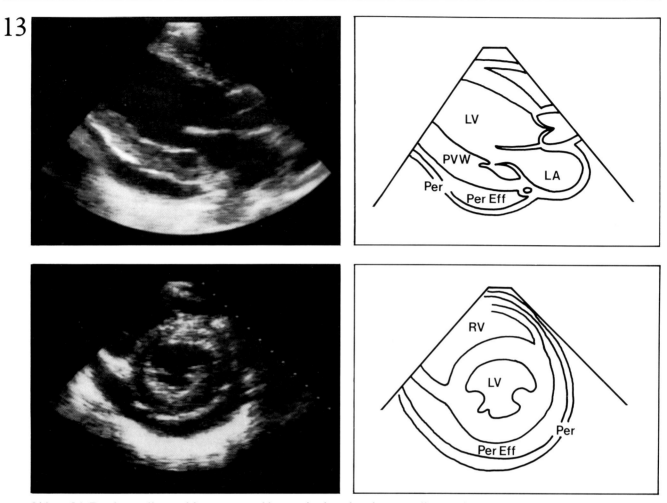

[Above] 2-D echocardiographic parasternal long axis view showing a small posterior pericardial effusion. [Below] 2-D echocardiographic parasternal short axis view showing a moderate pericardial effusion. The uneven distribution of the fluid can be seen in both views.

Chapter 7.

Miscellaneous Cardiac Conditions

Abbreviations

a	Anterior	LA	Left Atrium	p	Posterior
AP	Antero-Posterior	LL	Left Lateral	PA	Postero-Anterior
CW	Chest Wall	LV	Left Ventricle	RA	Right Atrium
Eff	Effusion	MV	Mitral Valve	RL	Right Lateral
IVS	Interventricular Septum	MVL	Mitral Valve Leaflet	RV	Right Ventricle

Pathology

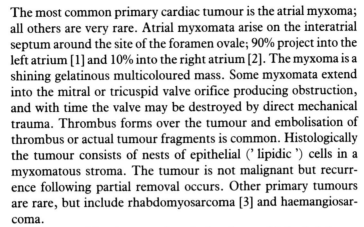

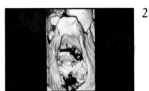

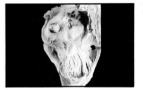

The most common primary cardiac tumour is the atrial myxoma; all others are very rare. Atrial myxomata arise on the interatrial septum around the site of the foramen ovale; 90% project into the left atrium [1] and 10% into the right atrium [2]. The myxoma is a shining gelatinous multicoloured mass. Some myxomata extend into the mitral or tricuspid valve orifice producing obstruction, and with time the valve may be destroyed by direct mechanical trauma. Thrombus forms over the tumour and embolisation of thrombus or actual tumour fragments is common. Histologically the tumour consists of nests of epithelial (' lipidic ') cells in a myxomatous stroma. The tumour is not malignant but recurrence following partial removal occurs. Other primary tumours are rare, but include rhabdomyosarcoma [3] and haemangiosarcoma.

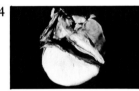

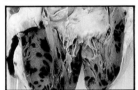

Children with tuberose sclerosis develop multiple rhabdomyomata consisting of large clear cells often interpreted as being masses of Purkinje cells. Occasionally isolated masses of fibrous tissue (fibromata or rhabdomyomata) are found in otherwise normal children [4].

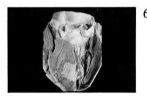

Secondary cardiac tumours are more common than primary neoplasms. Multiple small nodules may occur throughout the myocardium in carcinoma of the breast, malignant melanoma [5]or bronchial tumours. More rarely, single large tumour deposits occur [6]. Occasionally, renal carcinoma or hepatoma spreads to the right atrium via the vena cava, or bronchial carcinoma may spread to the left atrium via the pulmonary veins.

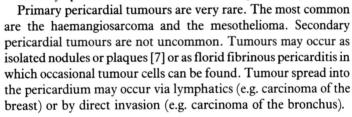

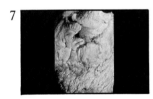

Primary pericardial tumours are very rare. The most common are the haemangiosarcoma and the mesothelioma. Secondary pericardial tumours are not uncommon. Tumours may occur as isolated nodules or plaques [7] or as florid fibrinous pericarditis in which occasional tumour cells can be found. Tumour spread into the pericardium may occur via lymphatics (e.g. carcinoma of the breast) or by direct invasion (e.g. carcinoma of the bronchus).

Presentation

Symptoms

Any cardiac tumour may present with a non-specific illness including a pyrexia and a high ESR. Tumours on the left side of the heart may present with single or multiple systemic emboli. Left atrial myxoma often presents with features indistinguishable from mitral valve disease. Similarly, right atrial myxomata mimic tricuspid valve disease and may present with embolism into the pulmonary circulation. Intermittent obstruction of the atrioventricular valves may result in syncope.

Signs

The physical signs of a left atrial myxoma may be indistinguishable from those of rheumatic mitral valve disease in sinus rhythm, including the same auscultatory features and the signs of pulmonary hypertension. Occasionally, a characteristic tumour 'plop' may distinguish left atrial myxoma from rheumatic mitral valve disease. Similarly, right atrial myxoma will closely mimic the physical signs of tricuspid valve disease.

Tumours involving the pericardium may present as a pericardial effusion or as cardiac tamponade. Where tumours extensively involve cardiac muscle the clinical features will be those of a restrictive cardiomyopathy.

Investigations

Radiology

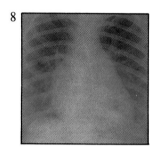

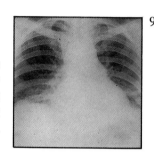

In left atrial myxoma, the chest x-ray may be normal or the appearances may reflect mitral valve obstruction with pulmonary venous hypertension [8]. With a right atrial myxoma the chest radiograph may show evidence of pulmonary infarcts - the result of tumour emboli [9]. An increased cardiac silhouette may be seen if there is a pericardial effusion.

Electrocardiography

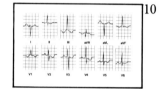

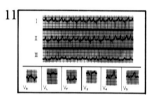

In left atrial myxoma obstructing the mitral valve, the electrocardiogram usually shows left atrial enlargement and may additionally show right ventricular hypertrophy [10] reflecting severe pulmonary hypertension. In right atrial myxoma obstructing the tricuspid valve, the electrocardiogram may show right atrial enlargement [11]. When a pericardial effusion is present, non specific ST-T changes and low voltage QRS complexes may be seen.

Echocardiography

Mobile tumours in the left atrium produce very characteristic echo recordings, which are diagnostic of the condition and preclude the need for further investigation.

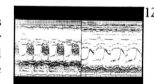

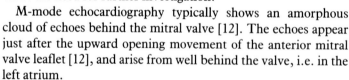

M-mode echocardiography typically shows an amorphous cloud of echoes behind the mitral valve [12]. The echoes appear just after the upward opening movement of the anterior mitral valve leaflet [12], and arise from well behind the valve, i.e. in the left atrium.

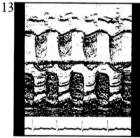

If the tumour is very mobile, it descends through the mitral orifice into the left ventricle during diastole, and returns to the left atrium during systole [13]. In other cases, the tumour stays mainly within the left atrium, and the echoes are only seen behind the mitral valve.

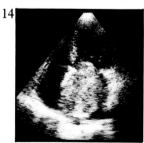

Two-dimensional echocardiography is an ideal technique for visualizing tumours within either atrium directly [14]. The mobility of an atrial myxoma usually enables it to be distinguished from the static thrombus. However, even large thrombi may not be seen at all since generally thrombus has the same echocardiographic appearance as blood.

No specific appearances are associated with intramural cardiac tumours, but any localized thickening of one of the chamber walls should raise the possibility of a tumour.

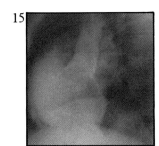

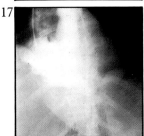

Cardiac Catheterization and Angiography

In patients with atrial myxomata the haemodynamics may reflect obstruction of the atrioventricular valves. Although rarely necessary for diagnostic purposes, particularly with the development of 2-D echocardiography, angiography when performed may show filling defects in the atria [15,16].

Where tumours involve the myocardium the haemodynamics may mimic restrictive cardiomyopathy while angiography may reveal encroachment on normal cardiac chambers [17]. Sometimes distortion of the normal coronary arterial pattern or even a pathological tumour circulation may be seen.

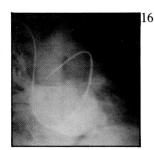

1 Left atrial myxoma. The tumour extends down into the mitral valve. Fibrous thickening is seen on the anterior cusp of the valve due to mechanical trauma from the tumour mass.

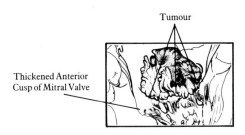

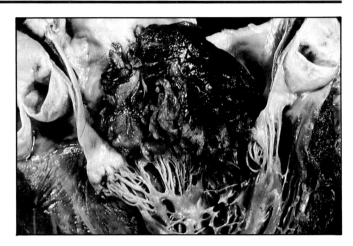

2 Right atrial myxoma. The tumour is a lobulated mass filling the cavity.

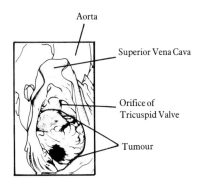

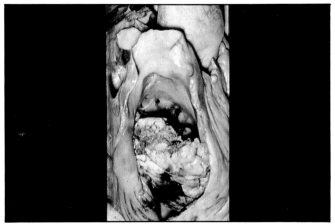

3 Rhabdomyosarcoma in the atrial septum. The right atrium is opened to show the bulging tumour mass which occupies the septum.

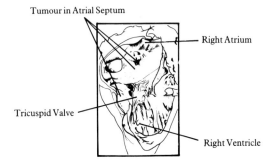

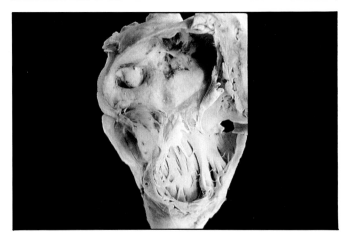

4 Right ventricular rhabdomyoma. A large solid white mass of tumour replaces most of the normal ventricular muscle.

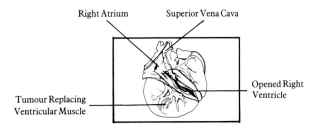

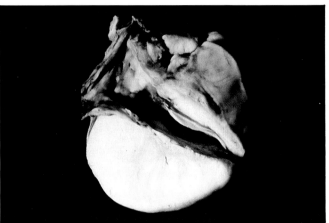

5 Secondary deposits of tumour in the heart. Multiple black deposits are seen in the myocardium secondary to malignant melanoma of the skin.

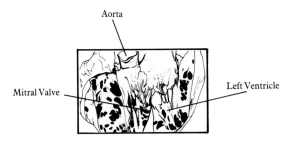

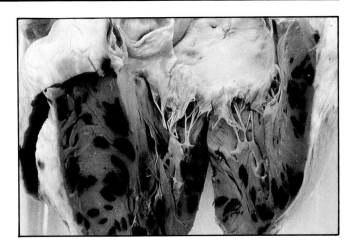

6 Single deposit of secondary carcinoma in the heart. The large tumour mass lies in the interventricular septum. The primary tumour site was in the kidney.

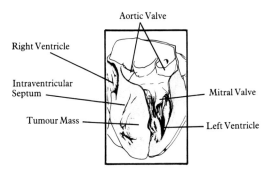

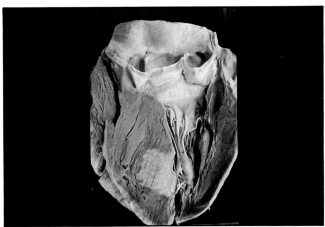

7 Secondary pericardial tumour. The pericardial cavity is opened to show the wide dissemination of tumour on the visceral pericardium of the right ventricle.

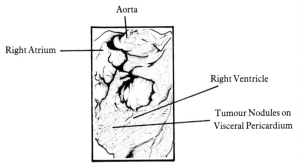

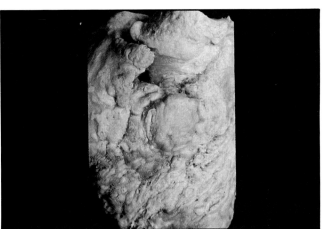

8 Chest radiograph in left atrial myxoma showing slight cardiac enlargement, prominent left atrial appendix and upper zone vessel dilatation indistinguishable from mitral valve disease.

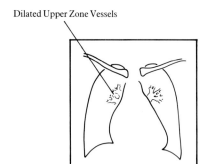

Dilated Upper Zone Vessels

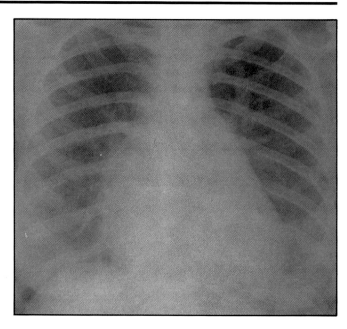

9 Chest radiograph in right atrial myxoma showing pulmonary infarcts in the left lung field.

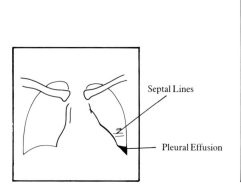

Septal Lines

Pleural Effusion

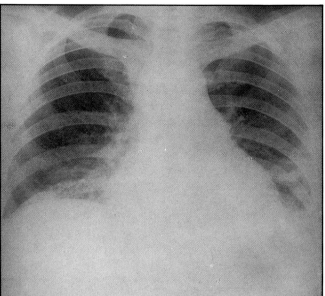

10

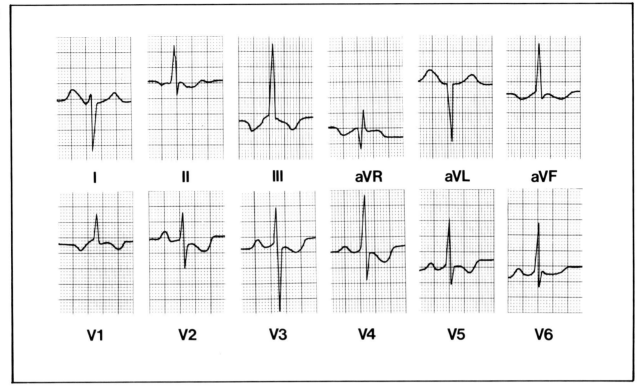

Electrocardiogram of a patient showing broad P wave of left atrial enlargement, with widespread T-wave inversion, dominant R wave in V_1 with deep S wave in V_5 indicating right ventricular hypertrophy.

11

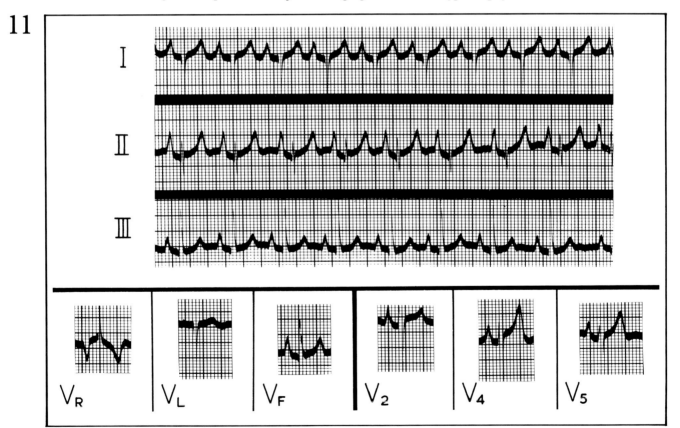

Electrocardiogram with tall P waves in lead II indicating right atrial enlargement.

12

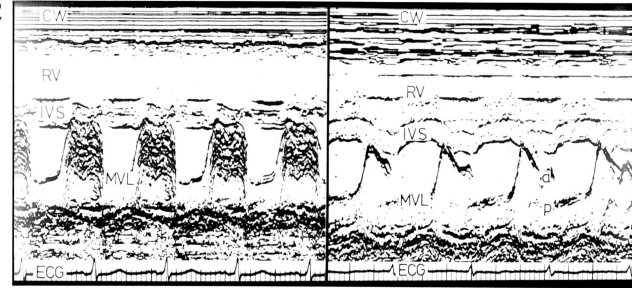

Echocardiogram of a left atrial myxoma. There is a short interval between mitral valve opening and the appearance of the tumour echoes [left]. After surgical removal of the myxoma, a normal mitral valve is seen [right].

13

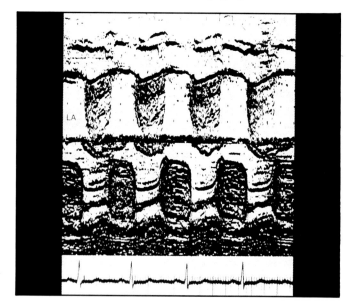

Echocardiogram of a mobile tumour seen in the left atrium during systole [top] and moving into the left ventricle behind the mitral valve during diastole [bottom]. The two recordings have been aligned using the electrocardiogram as a timing reference.

14

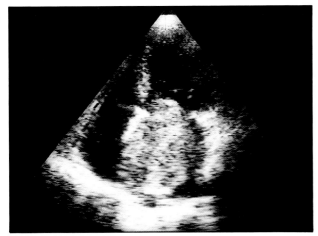

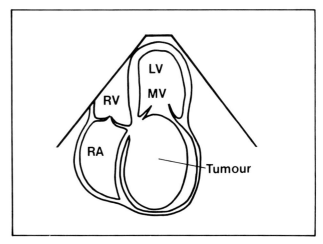

2-D echocardiographic apical four-chamber view showing a very large mass filling the left atrium. On the moving image it showed a rocking motion, indicating attachment to the interatrial septum behind the mitral valve. The mass was shown to be a myxoma at surgery.

15 Right atrial angiogram (lateral projection) showing large filling defect caused by myxoma.

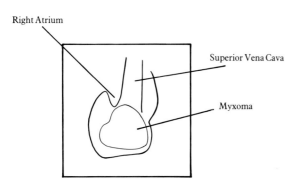

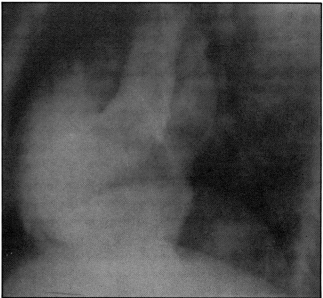

16 Pulmonary arteriogram showing pulmonary venous phase. The left atrium contains an extensive filling defect due to myxoma.

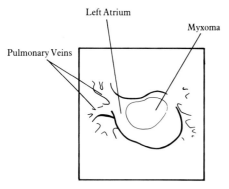

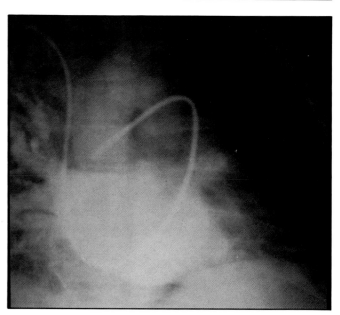

17 Right atrial angiogram showing gross distortion of the normal cavity due to infiltration of the right atrial wall by tumour.

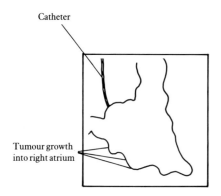

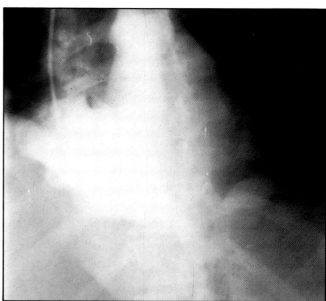

Pulmonary hypertension may occur in patients with:

1) an elevated pulmonary venous pressure due to abnormalities in the left heart such as mitral stenosis, left atrial myxoma, cor triatriatum and left ventricular disease of any aetiology;

2) increased pulmonary blood flow from a left to right intra or extra-cardiac shunt such as ventricular septal defect, atrial septal defect or persistent ductus arteriosus;

3) intra or extra-cardiac shunts with pulmonary vascular disease (Eisenmenger syndrome).

These conditions will be dealt with in their relevant sections. This section will deal with other causes:

4) pulmonary embolic disease;

5) chronic hypoxic conditions including diseases of lung parenchyma and high altitude;

6) idiopathic (primary) pulmonary hypertension.

Pathology

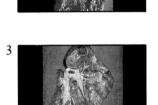

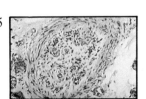

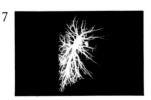

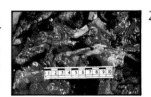

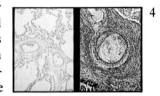

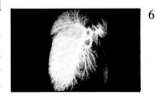

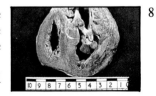

Pulmonary embolism may be massive or minor, acute or chronic. Acute pulmonary embolism usually results from the passage of thrombus originating in a systemic vein [1] through the right side of the heart and lodging in the pulmonary arteries [2]. If the embolism is massive, the right ventricle becomes acutely dilated. If the embolism is minor a pulmonary infarct may develop [3].

Chronic thrombo-embolic disease results in severe pulmonary hypertension due to long-standing obstruction to right ventricular outflow. Histologically, the pulmonary arteries show mild medial hypertrophy, eccentric intimal fibrosis and intraluminal fibrous septa, an appearance which distinguishes this condition from primary pulmonary hypertension. Chronic hypoxia due to parenchymal lung disease or living at high altitude may also cause changes in pulmonary arterioles with secondary pulmonary hypertension. The histological changes include eccentric intimal fibrosis with longitudinal muscle bundles in the intima.

Some cases of pulmonary hypertension are due to primary disease of the small pulmonary arterioles [4,5] the cause of which is unknown. Histologically, there is medial hypertrophy, concentric and laminary intimal fibrosis, with medial fibrinoid necrosis with or without arteritis and the so-called 'plexiform' lesion. Similar histological appearances may be seen in patients with the Eisenmenger syndrome. There is an overall decrease in the number of pulmonary arteries with reduction of calibre of the peripheral vessels [6,7].

All cases of long standing severe pulmonary hypertension will result in right ventricular hypertrophy [8].

Presentation

Symptoms

Acute massive pulmonary embolism presents with the features of sudden reduction in cardiac output (collapse and circulatory arrest). Sudden severe breathlessness is another common presentation. Pleuritic chest pain is usually not a feature of acute massive embolism, but there may have been prior episodes of pleurisy due to minor pulmonary embolism. Acute minor embolism usually results in pulmonary infarction with pleurisy and/or haemoptysis being the main features. Usually there is a clear predisposing factor for the development of thrombo-embolism such as surgery, trauma, bed rest, neoplastic disease or severe generalised disease. Chronic pulmonary thrombo-embolic disease presents with the features of severe pulmonary hypertension (exertional dyspnoea or syncope sometimes with repetitive episodes of pleurisy and haemoptysis).

If pulmonary hypertension is due to chronic parenchymal lung disease the symptomatology will be dominated by the respiratory abnormality.

Idiopathic (primary) pulmonary hypertension is most frequently seen in young women. The presentation is insidious with increasing breathlessness, occasionally exertional syncope and sometimes haemoptysis. Angina–like chest pain sometimes occurs.

Signs

Massive pulmonary embolism will result in the physical signs of a low cardiac output (peripheral vasoconstriction, hypotension, sinus tachycardia, oliguria, cerebral confusion) and right ventricular failure (elevation of jugular venous pressure, and a gallop rhythm at the left sternal edge). Minor pulmonary embolism causing pulmonary infarction has physical signs confined to the respiratory system such as a pleural rub, lobar collapse or consolidation or a pleural effusion.

Severe pulmonary hypertension as occurs in long-standing hypoxic lung disease, chronic thrombo-embolic disease or of idiopathic aetiology gives rise to a loud pulmonary component of the second heart sound usually with normal respiratory variation in the width of splitting. There may be palpable right ventricular hypertrophy. The jugular venous pulse may either show abnormal dominance of the 'a' wave or a frank rise in venous pressure with or without obvious tricuspid regurgitation if there is additional right ventricular failure. Hepatic engorgement and fluid retention characterised by peripheral oedema and ascites may be present. Respiratory failure is often present when the cause is long-standing parenchymal lung disease.

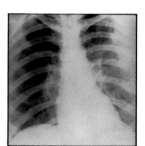

9

Investigations

Radiology

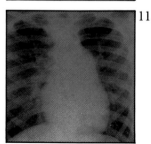

11

In acute massive pulmonary embolism the chest radiograph shows areas of oligaemia due to patchy reduction in blood flow interspersed with areas of compensatory hyperaemia [9]. The central pulmonary arteries are not enlarged. In minor pulmonary embolism the chest x-ray may be normal or show features consistent with pulmonary infarction (lobar collapse/consolidation with or without pleural effusion) [10].

In primary pulmonary hypertension the heart and central pulmonary arteries are characteristically enlarged in a non-specific way and the peripheral vessels diffusely reduced in size [11].

PULMONARY EMBOLIC/VASCULAR DISEASE

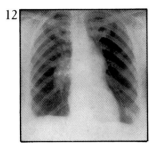

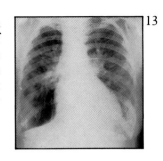

Thrombo-embolic pulmonary hypertension is distinguished from primary pulmonary hypertension by an irregular distribution of the vascular obliteration in the lungs [12]. In parenchymatous lung disease causing chronic pulmonary hypertension the nature of the lung disease may be identified by specific appearances, but the cardiovascular changes are similar to those seen in pulmonary hypertension from other causes [13].

Electrocardiography

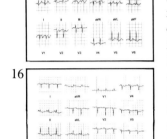

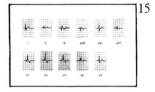

In acute massive pulmonary embolism, the electrocardiogram may show a $S_1Q_3T_3$ pattern [14], right bundle branch block [15], or right ventricular 'strain' with T wave inversion over the anterior precordial leads [14]. In minor pulmonary embolism the ECG is normal. In chronic pulmonary hypertension from any cause, the electrocardiogram usually reflects the right ventricular hypertrophy with right axis deviation, right atrial enlargement and T wave inversion over the right ventricle (anterior precordial leads). The R wave is dominant in lead V_1 and S wave dominant in V_5 [16].

Arterial blood gases

Blood gases in massive pulmonary embolism usually show hypoxia and hypocapnia; in minor pulmonary embolism the gases will be normal. In chronic pulmonary hypertension due to lung disease it is likely there will be hypoxia and hypercapnia; in idiopathic and chronic thrombo-embolic pulmonary hypertension there will be hypoxia.

Nuclear Techniques

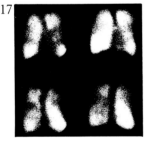

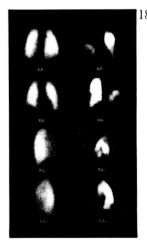

Simultaneous ventilation (using krypton-81m or xenon) and perfusion scans (using technetium-99m labelled macroaggregated albumin) will permit distinction between primary lung pathology e.g. emphysema (matched ventilation-perfusion defects), and pulmonary vascular disease due to pulmonary embolism (where the ventilation scan is normal but there are variable defects of perfusion [17,18]).

Echocardiography

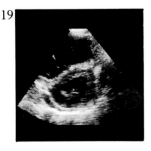

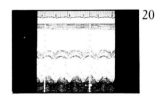

Long-standing severe pulmonary hypertension gives rise to right ventricular hypertrophy and dilatation and secondary right atrial dilatation. These features may be identified by echocardiography [19]. The M-mode echocardiogram usually shows reversed septal motion [20]. A key role of the echocardiogram is to eliminate left heart abnormalities such as mitral valve disease, left atrial myxoma and left ventricular disease as causes of pulmonary hypertension.

Cardiac Catheterization and Angiography

In acute massive pulmonary embolism there is only moderate elevation of pulmonary artery pressure distinguishing this condi-

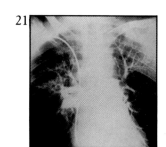

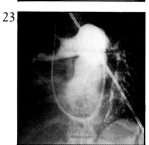

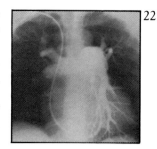

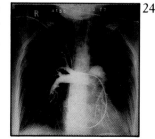

tion from chronic thromboembolic disease where the pulmonary artery pressures are usually much higher. In minor pulmonary embolism the pulmonary artery pressure is normal.

In massive pulmonary embolism the angiogram shows obstruction to a major portion of the total pulmonary arterial bed [21]. In chronic thrombo-embolic pulmonary hypertension the pulmonary trunk is enlarged and there is an asymmetric obliteration of pulmonary vessels, those unaffected by thrombus being tortuous and dilated [22]. There is a convex leading-edge to contrast-filled vessels obstructed by thrombus [22] unlike the concave leading-edge in acute embolism [23]. In primary (idiopathic) pulmonary hypertension the pulmonary vasculature shows symmetrical peripheral pruning [24].

1 Thrombus in the femoral vein.

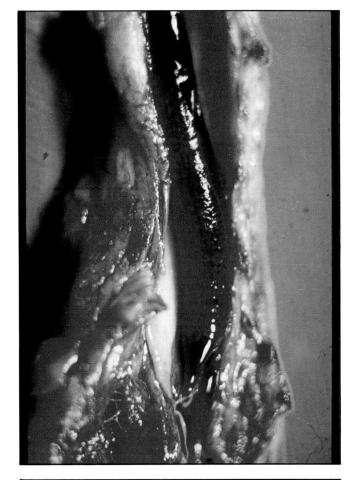

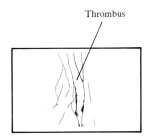

Thrombus

2 Large saddle embolus is seen astride both right and left pulmonary arteries.

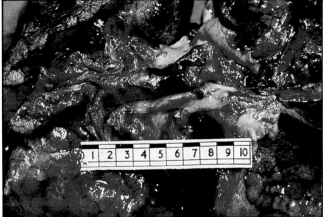

Right Pulmonary Artery

Left Pulmonary Artery

Embolus

3 Minor pulmonary embolism in the upper lobe arteries resulting in infarction of the lung.

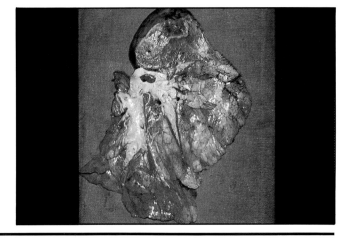

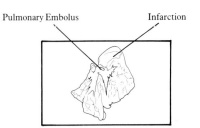

Pulmonary Embolus

Infarction

4 Normal pulmonary arteries (left panel) compared with small pulmonary artery affected by intimal fibrosis as a consequence of severe primary pulmonary hypertension (right panel).

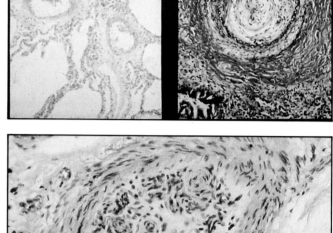

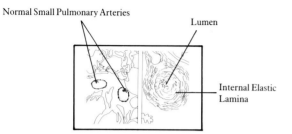

Normal Small Pulmonary Arteries

Lumen

Internal Elastic Lamina

5 Complex angiomatoid lesions in small pulmonary arteries in primary pulmonary hypertension.

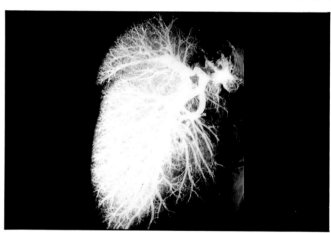

Small Vascular Spaces

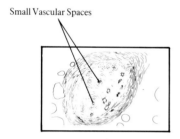

6 Normal post-mortem pulmonary arteriogram.

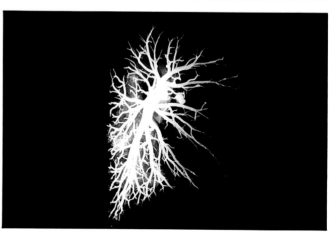

Filling of Peripheral Vessels

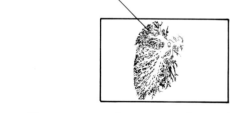

7 Post-mortem pulmonary arteriogram in primary pulmonary hypertension.

Peripheral 'Pruning'

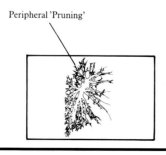

8   Gross right ventricular hypertrophy secondary to primary pulmonary hypertension. The right ventricular wall thickness and size greatly exceed those of the left ventricle.

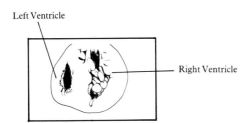

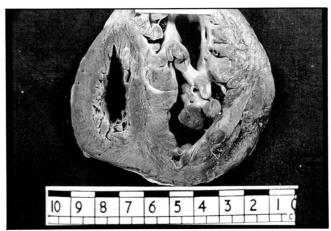

9   Chest radiograph of acute massive pulmonary embolism showing oligaemia in the right lung with compensatory hyperaemia in the left lung.

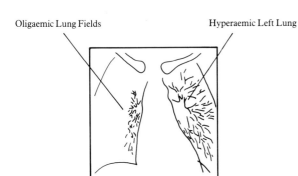

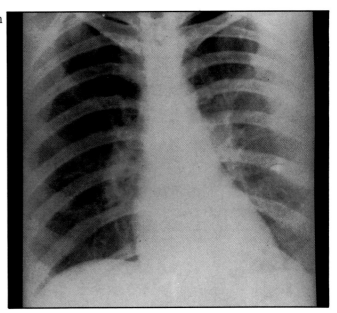

10 Chest radiograph of pulmonary infarction. Note shadow at right lung base and elevated right hemidiaphragm.

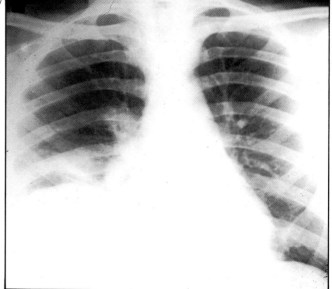

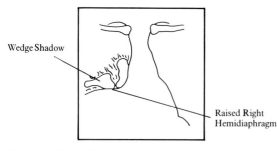

Wedge Shadow

Raised Right Hemidiaphragm

11 Chest radiograph of primary pulmonary hypertension showing large central pulmonary arteries and symmetrical reduction in peripheral vessel size.

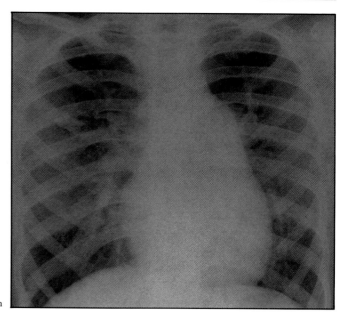

Large Central Arteries

Symmetrical Peripheral Reduction

12 Chest radiograph in thrombo-embolic pulmonary hypertension showing large pulmonary trunk and right hilar artery. The left lung is oligaemic.

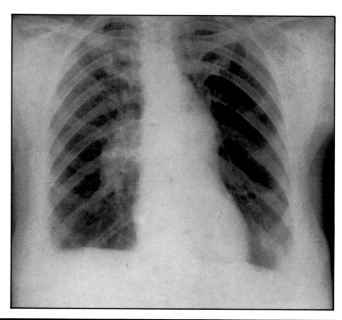

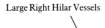
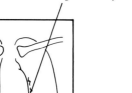

Large Right Hilar Vessels

Large Pulmonary Trunk

13 Chest radiograph in obstructive airway disease with cor pulmonale showing large heart and hilar arteries with irregular pulmonary vascular obliteration.

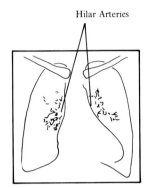

Hilar Arteries

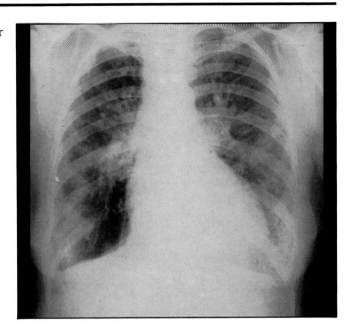

PULMONARY EMBOLIC/VASCULAR DISEASE   Electrocardiography

14

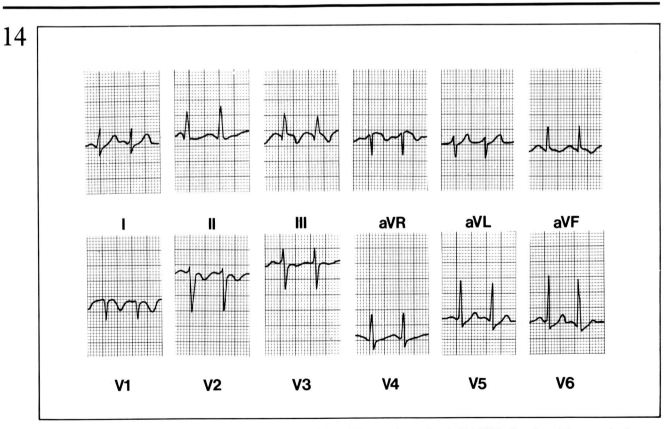

Electrocardiogram showing $S_1Q_3T_3$ pattern and additional T-wave inversion in V1-V3 indicating right ventricular strain.

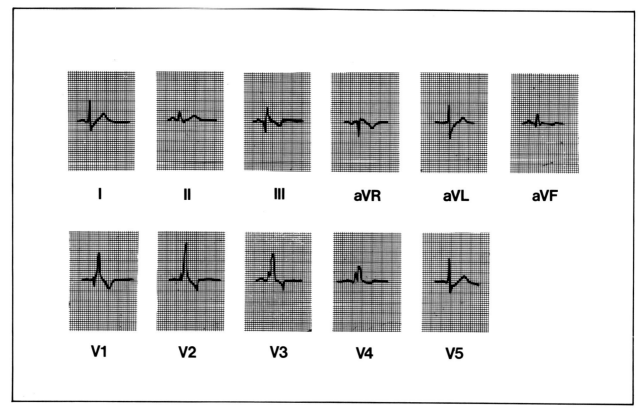

Electrocardiogram showing right bundle branch block.

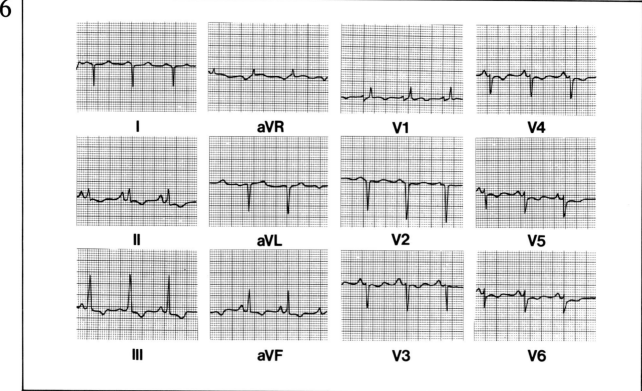

Electrocardiogram showing 'P' pulmonale, right axis deviation and right ventricular hypertrophy.

17 Ventilation [left panel] and perfusion [right panel] lung scans in chronic obstructive airways disease showing matched defects.

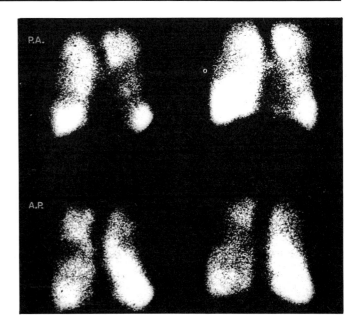

18 Ventilation [left panel] and perfusion [right panel] lung scans in pulmonary embolic disease, showing normal ventilation but multiple perfusion defects.

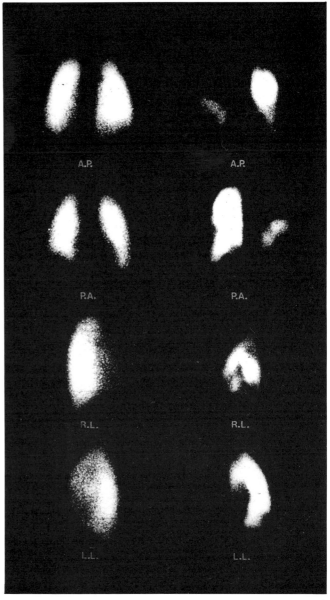

19

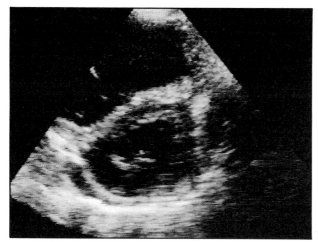 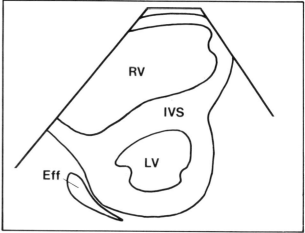

2-D echocardiographic parasternal short axis view of pulmonary hypertension secondary to chronic obstructive airways disease. The right ventricle is enlarged and the left ventricle is small. The interventricular septum is less curved than normal, giving the left ventricle a flattened appearance.

20

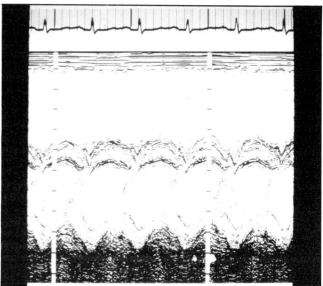

M-mode echocardiogram showing reversed septal motion in a patient with pulmonary hypertension.

21 Pulmonary arteriogram in acute massive pulmonary embolism showing involvement of more than 50% of the major pulmonary arteries.

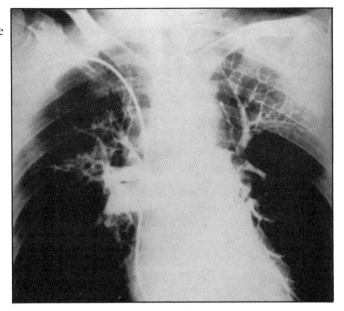

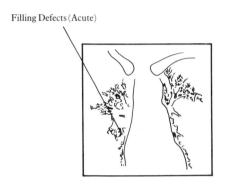

Filling Defects (Acute)

22 Pulmonary arteriogram in chronic thromboembolic pulmonary hypertension. The pulmonary trunk is dilated, and vessels unaffected by thrombus are dilated and tortuous.

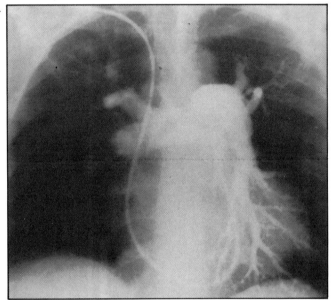

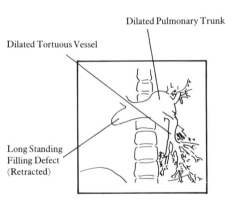

Dilated Pulmonary Trunk

Dilated Tortuous Vessel

Long Standing Filling Defect (Retracted)

23 Pulmonary arteriogram in acute massive pulmonary embolism showing acute thrombus in right pulmonary artery causing a concave leading edge.

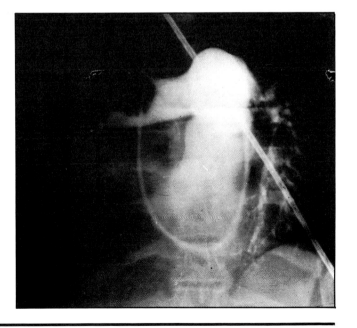

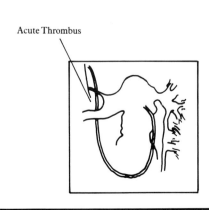

Acute Thrombus

24 Pulmonary arteriogram in primary pulmonary
hypertension showing peripheral arterial pruning.

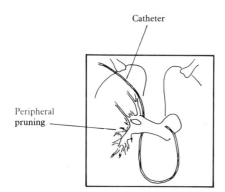

Catheter

Peripheral
pruning

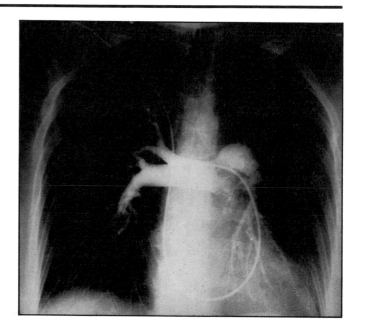

INDEX

INDEX

in pulmonary embolic/vascular disease, 274, 279

Pulmonary hypertension *see also* Pulmonary embolic/vascular disease
  in atrial septal defect, 178-179, 182
  with cardiac tumours, 264
  in coarctation of the aorta, 219, 222
  in dilated cardiomyopathy, 227, 229
  in heart failure, 43-45, 50-53
  in hypertrophic cardiomyopathy, 237, 241
  in ischaemic heart disease, 4, 7
  in mitral regurgitation, 120
  in persistent ductus arteriosus, 199
  in rheumatic mitral valve disease, 108-109
  in ventricular septal defect, 188-190, 193, 195

Pulmonary infarction
  with cardiac tumours, 264, 268
  in pulmonary embolic/vascular disease, 273-274, 277, 280

Pulmonary infundibular stenosis *see also* Pulmonary stenosis
  Fallot's tetralogy, 212-218

Pulmonary oedema
  in aortic regurgitation, 152, 157
  in aortic stenosis, 138
  in dilated cardiomyopathy, 227
  in heart failure, 43-44, 51-53
  in hypertension, 94
  in ischaemic heart disease, 5, 12
  in mitral regurgitation, 120
  in restrictive cardiomyopathy, 246

Pulmonary oligaemia
  in pulmonary embolic/vascular disease, 274, 279-280
  in pulmonary stenosis, 205
  in tricuspid valve disease, 165, 168

Pulmonary plethora
  in atrial septal defect, 178, 182-183
  in persistent ductus arteriosus, 198, 200
  in ventricular septal defect, 189, 193

Pulmonary stenosis, 205-211
  cardiac catheterization and angiography, 206, 211
  echocardiography, 206, 210
  electrocardiography, 206, 209
  pathology, 205, 207
  radiology, 205, 208
  signs, 205
  symptoms, 205

Pulmonary valve calcification
  in pulmonary stenosis, 205

Pulmonary valve stenosis *see also* Pulmonary stenosis
  Fallot's tetralogy, 212-218
  with tricuspid valve disease, 173

Pulmonary vascular resistance
  in persistent ductus arteriosus, 199
  in rheumatic mitral valve disease, 109

Pulmonary vessels
  in atrial septal defect, 178-179, 181-183
  in aortic stenosis, 134, 139
  with cardiac tumours, 268
  in dilated cardiomyopathy, 227, 229
  in Fallot's tetralogy, 215
  in hypertension, 84, 99
  in hypertrophic cardiomyopathy, 237, 241
  in mitral regurgitation, 120, 124
  in persistent ductus arteriosus, 198-201

in pulmonary embolic/vascular disease, 274, 276, 280-281, 285
  in pulmonary stenosis, 205-207, 211
  in rheumatic mitral valve disease, 108, 112, 114
  in ventricular septal defect, 189, 193

Pulmonary vessel obliteration
  in pulmonary embolic/vascular disease, 275-276, 285

Pulmonary vessel obstruction
  in pulmonary embolic/vascular disease, 276, 285

Pulmonary vessel peripheral pruning
  in pulmonary embolic/vascular disease, 276, 286

Purulent pericarditis, 252, 254

Pyelonephritis
  in hypertension, 80, 84-85, 88, 100

Q wave changes
  in dilated cardiomyopathy, 227, 231
  in heart failure, 54, 55, 57
  in ischaemic heart disease, 5, 18-22
  in hypertrophic cardiomyopathy, 237, 242

QR wave abnormalities
  in hypertrophic cardiomyopathy, 237

QRS complex abnormalities
  with cardiac tumours, 264
  in coarctation of the aorta, 223
  in hypertrophic cardiomyopathy, 237, 242

R wave abnormalities
  in aortic regurgitation, 152, 157
  in aortic stenosis, 140
  with cardiac tumours, 269
  in heart failure, 55, 57
  in hypertension, 84, 98
  in ischaemic heart disease, 20
  in persistent ductus arteriosus, 199, 202
  in pulmonary embolic/vascular disease, 275
  in pulmonary stenosis, 209
  in rheumatic mitral valve disease, 109, 115
  in ventricular septal defect, 189, 194

Radiology *see also* Renal radiology
  aortic regurgitation, 152, 156-157
  aortic stenosis, 133-134, 138-139
  atrial septal defect, 178, 181-183
  cardiac tumours, 264, 268
  coarctation of the aorta, 219-220, 222
  dilated cardiomyopathy, 227, 229
  Fallot's tetralogy, 212, 215
  heart failure, 44, 50-54
  hypertension, 84, 99
  hypertrophic cardiomyopathy, 237, 240-241
  ischaemic heart disease, 4-5, 12-13
  mitral regurgitation (non-rheumatic), 120, 123-124
  pericardial disease, 253, 255-256
  persistent ductus arteriosus, 198-201
  pulmonary embolic/vascular disease, 274-275, 279-281
  pulmonary stenosis, 205, 208
  restrictive cardiomyopathy, 246-247, 249
  rheumatic mitral valve disease, 108, 111-114
  tricuspid valve disease, 165, 168-169
  ventricular septal defect, 189, 193

Radionuclide ventriculography

in heart failure, 46, 62-64
  in ischaemic heart disease, 6, 28-30

Red cell casts
  in hypertension, 84, 98

Renal angiography
  hypertension, 85, 100

Renal artery stenosis
  in hypertension, 85-87, 99-100

Renal failure
  in hypertension, 83

Renal haemorrhage
  in hypertension, 83, 96

Renal hypertension
  investigations, 84-86
  pathology, 80

Renal infarction
  in hypertension, 83

Renal ischaemia
  in hypertension, 80

Renal radiology
  hypertension, 84-85, 99-101

Renal scarring
  in hypertension, 83

Renal size
  in hypertension, 83, 85, 96

Restrictive cardiomyopathy, 246-251
  cardiac catheterization and angiography, 247, 251
  echocardiography, 247, 250
  electrocardiography, 247
  in heart failure, 43, 45, 47
  pathology, 246, 248
  radiology, 246-247, 249
  signs, 246
  symptoms, 246

Retinopathy
  in hypertension, 84, 97

Rheumatic aortic incompetence
  in aortic regurgitation, 151, 154

Rheumatic mitral valve disease, 107-118
  cardiac catheterization and angiography, 109, 118
  echocardiography, 109, 115-117
  electrocardiography, 109, 115
  pathology, 107, 110-111
  radiology, 108, 111-114
  signs, 108
  symptoms, 107-108

Rheumatic tricuspid valve disease, 164-165, 167-168
  with aortic and mitral valve disease, 164-166, 169, 172

Rheumatoid disease
  in pericardial disease, 252

Rib notching
  in coarctation of the aorta, 84, 99, 220, 222

Right atrial dilatation
  in atrial septal defect, 178
  in pulmonary embolic/vascular disease, 275

Right atrial enlargement
  with cardiac tumours, 264
  in pulmonary embolic/vascular disease, 275
  in pulmonary stenosis, 206
  in tricuspid valve disease, 165-166, 168-169, 173

Right atrial filling defect with cardiac tumours, 265, 271

Right atrial hypertrophy
  in Fallot's tetralogy, 212
  in tricuspid valve disease, 165, 170

Right axis deviation

INDEX

in restrictive cardiomyopathy,
247, 251
in tricuspid valve disease, 166
T wave abnormalities
in aortic stenosis, 134
with cardiac tumours, 269
in hypertension, 84, 98
in hypertrophic cardiomyopathy,
237
in ischaemic heart disease, 18-21
in pericardial disease, 253, 257
in persistent ductus arteriosus,
199, 202
in pulmonary embolic/vascular
disease, 275, 281
in pulmonary stenosis, 209
in restrictive cardiomyopathy, 247
in ventricular septal defect, 194
Tricuspid valve disease, 164-173
cardiac catheterization and
angiography, 166, 172-173
echocardiography, 165-166,
170-172
electrocardiography, 165, 169-170
with mitral valve disease, 109
pathology, 164, 167
radiology, 165, 168-169
signs, 164-165
symptoms, 164
Tricuspid valve movement

in tricuspid valve disease,
165-166, 171
Tricuspid valve obstruction
with cardiac tumours, 263-264
Tricuspid valve stenosis, 165,
167-168, 171
Tuberculosis
and pericardial disease, 252

Ultrasonic scanning
hypertension, 85, 102
Uraemic pericarditis, 252

Vascular system
in hypertension, 81-82, 92-93
Vasodilatation
in hypertension, 83
Vegetations on valves
in aortic regurgitation, 152,
154, 159-160
in mitral regurgitation, 120,
122, 128
in rheumatic mitral valve disease,
107, 110
Ventilation scans
in pulmonary embolic/vascular
disease, 275, 283
Ventricular fibrillation
in hypertrophic cardiomyopathy,
236
in restrictive cardiomyopathy, 246

Ventricular septal defect, 188-197
cardiac catheterization and
angiography, 190, 197
echocardiography, 189-190, 195-196
electrocardiography, 189, 194
Fallot's tetralogy, 212-218
in hypertension, 91
in ischaemic heart disease, 10,
12-13, 33
pathology, 188, 191-192
in pulmonary stenosis, 205
radiology, 189, 193
signs, 188-189
symptoms, 188
Ventricular tachycardia
in heart failure, 57-58
Viral infection
and dilated cardiomyopathy, 227
and pericardial disease, 252, 254

Wall movement
in dilated cardiomyopathy,
228, 231
in heart failure, 46, 64
in pericardial disease, 253
Wilm's tumour
and hypertension, 80, 88
Wolff-Parkinson-White syndrome
in hypertrophic cardiomyopathy,
237